Forty Years Stoned

Forty Years Stoned

a journalist's romance

TOM HUTH

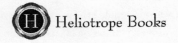
Heliotrope Books

New York

If you expect it will get you high,
you're already halfway there.

This tale is dedicated to Holly Young Huth,
the love of my life and my partner in adventure—
a woman who has made an eloquent performance art
out of her living, and her dying.

Table of Contents

Prelude

October, 1996

Holly and I are lying in bed on a Sunday afternoon in our lost-and-found ghost town in the Colorado Rockies. We're watching a Denver Broncos game, or at least I am. My arm is around her shoulder; her head is tucked under my chin. Sundays are the days that we snuggle in: first having coffee with Charles Kuralt, then sharing a pipeful, then moving straight on to making whoopee. Is it wrong to be so scheduled? On Sundays I don't care.

The Broncos are playing the Kansas City Chiefs. We have the ball when I notice that Holly is...is she crying?

I cock my head to have a look. "Are you crying?"

It's not the most receptive tone of voice. I should encourage her; she hardly ever cries. But the Broncos are driving. Elway dropping back to pass...

I venture, "What's the problem?"

"Nothing."

Christ, was there a flag on that play?

"How come you're crying?"

No flag.

She blurts: "Something's wrong with me!"

Reflexively: "Nothing's wrong with you!"

"I can tell something's wrong."

DID HE FUMBLE?

"What is it?"

She doesn't answer. It's a lost opportunity: They've broken for a commercial.

As soon as the game comes back on then, she says: "You know in Costa Rica last winter how my fingers kind of fluttered when I was doing yoga?"

"Yeah...?"

DAMN! Chiefs' ball.

"It's happening more. You've noticed it yourself."

I protest, "It's just what your mother had, honey! You know her hands, when she got stressed?"

I hate to hear her worry about her health. When we watch the news, her ears will perk up at the latest medical scare. She's in fantastic shape at 52—robust, athletic. But she feels vulnerable to disease, whereas I'm oblivious to it. If you talk about getting sick, if you even think about it, aren't you inviting the sickness right in?

Okay, I get scared, too. Sometimes she reminds me of her mother, who was a nervous wreck of a hypochondriac. With my fears matched up against her fears, I invariably respond to any issues about bodily disintegration, either hers or mine, either past, present or future, with a breezy, "It'll probably be fine." And I take some measure of satisfaction that I am always right.

She sniffles, "I know it's not just what Mom had."

I hug her tighter, Mr. Empathy. The Chiefs settle for a field goal. My fears against her fears: like sets of opposing linemen. I figure that we can talk about it at halftime. But by then she's asleep, and I can't feel anything shaking inside.

Three months later she is diagnosed.

She has Parkinson's disease.

We walk out of the neurologist's sanctum, in silence. I schedule her next appointment. Six months from now.

"No urgency, I guess," I murmur.

She wonders, "Is that good?"

I force a laugh. "Who knows?"

We walk out to the hallway and wait for the elevator to come. What is there to say? Our eyes meet—a glance of acknowledgment, a rock-bottom recognition, a glimmer of understanding that somehow our lives are still moving ahead, from one breath to the next.

I ask, "Got your purse?"

She holds it out.

I'm taking care of her already.

We walk out of the medical center, and I look back to take in its corporate façade: this doomplex to which we've been sentenced to keep returning every six months for news that will keep getting worse and worse.

Plainly, I have no aptitude for helping another human being who's in any kind of serious need. But I've already left one wife. That won't be happening again.

Over the countless years which ensue, I will settle into the job of being Holly's caregiver. At first serving as her chauffeur and chaperon. Later, helping her stand up and sit down and get dressed. Still later, helping her walk. Bathing her. Wiping her. Watching her get weaker and weaker in body and mind.

Fortunately, we enjoy the love of our children and our friends. But we also draw immeasurable sustenance from a secret (or not so secret) habit which can elevate us one toke at a time above the drudgeries and distresses of our mortal fix. That is the story this book will tell.

I don't mean to trivialize what an awful disease we are dealing with. Parkinson's, unlike cancer, is a fight that everyone loses, day after endless day. It's not kind enough to kill, but lets you stick around to find out just what it feels like to keep giving up control of your once-agile body and your once-expert mind to the neuroterrorists who are dedicated to sapping you of every last sliver of independence, dignity and self-respect while stringing out the toll for fifteen or twenty or who knows how many years.

Smoking marijuana will never lift this spell. But it has often worked to distract Holly from her discomforts and anxieties. And, as this report from the front lines will amply document, dope has been especially generous to me by providing untold tens of thousands of sweet reprieves which continue to give me the pizzazz, at 74, to go deep into extra innings with her.

In 1999, two years after she is diagnosed, we buy a winter home in Santa Barbara, where growing old might feel a little easier than it does in the mountains.

While she still has the wherewithal to take a walk, I like to whisk her away in the middle of the day to a park or to the beach. As the new century wobbles on through the turmoil of 9/11 and the Bush and Obama years, our strolls keep getting slower and slower and shorter and shorter. Yet they give my comrade her only remaining glimpses of the outside world. Her curiosity is waning, and I'm determined to enhance each opportunity.

She prepares for our walk by fussing around in the bedroom. She might say, "I don't feel well enough to go out." I might suggest, "That's why you need to go out."

She totters downstairs. I coax her to pick out a hat. She stares into the mirror with the discerning eye of the New York fashion editor she once was. She tries another hat. I wait. I wait. Holly has taught me how to wait.

At last, when she's ready to walk out the door, I give her a single hit on a small wooden pipe.

I take a hit myself, thank you. Then I shepherd her out to the car, and as we drive away I look for signs that her focus is making that beneficent shift, from the inward to the outward, from the subjective to the wondrous other. She might remark, "Look at that bougainvillea!" At the beach, she might delight in the shapes of the stones.

It's that one-two punch that works: getting her out of the house, and letting the cannabis help to open her eyes. This vacation from uneasiness and self-regard can last for part of the walk, or all of it, or for the rest of the day. Except when, alas, it doesn't lift the veil at all.

My own relationship with the smoke is more devotional.

Pot is my co-pilot. Pot is my refresh button. Pot makes the familiar look new. It makes the mundane suddenly (if temporarily) fascinating. It makes the everyday feel like one-of-a-kind. Not all of the time, no. But enough of the time.

It relieves those burnt-out-caregiver blahs. It helps me blossom into a sunnier companion. It gives me something to say even if she can't muster a reply. It can embolden me to talk with her about difficult subjects, like death.

The caregiver longs for periods when no one wants him or needs him. When Holly sleeps in late, I have time alone to pursue my writing. When she lies down for a nap, I go for a walk. During these breaks, my perspective-enhancing drug can render certain random moments uncommonly exquisite and eventful. This slows down the clock—hell, it stops the clock—expanding the sense of how much time I have. What a gift it is for the incidental shut-in: to be able to conjure these daily illusions of unlimited space.

Dinnertime is another opportunity to renew myself and my commitment to the job. Holly was a superb cook in her day, a natural. Under our new division of labor (every job mine), I can resent having to cook, or I can enjoy it. So this has become a golden part of each day—helping milady get cozy on the couch upstairs, where she can snooze off or meditate, then tiptoeing down to the kitchen to carve a precious kingdom of solitude out of the early evening.

The recipe is simple. One heaping suck on the bong, and I'm baked. Then I can get lost (chop, chop, sizzle, sizzle) in the satisfactions of completing each chore and the free-range adventures of an untethered mind.

In a time of uncertainty for both of us, an ordinary meal can be something to celebrate. Here is one small but concrete victory over potential despair and disarray. I might not have the power to alter her ultimate outcome. But night after night I can dish up a reasonably healthy, relatively tasty dinner while still serving myself those side orders of whimsy and inspiration.

Just as there are different strains of marijuana, so there are different strains of stoners. You have your social smokers and your lone wolves, your couch potatoes and your future presidents, your stoner actors and athletes and surgeons and farmers and firefighters and welders and circuit-court judges and moms and dads. I am charting my own course, as a solid stoner helpmate: chronically chipper, mindlessly industrious, resilient on demand, fully rechargeable, easy to please, slow to take umbrage, inexplicably reliable and (of crucial importance) excellent at keeping myself amused for long stretches of downtime.

Highs in the '70s

1972
My Watergate Affair

This is the dawn of the Stoned Age, the time when I first start wanting to feel it every day—that alertness, that spaciousness, that all-consuming all-is-wellness.

What a year it is: 1972. Jane Fonda goes to North Vietnam and poses astride an anti-aircraft gun. Weatherman revolutionaries Bernadette Dohrn and Kathy Boudin set off bombs in ladies' rooms at the Capitol and the Pentagon. Angela Davis is found innocent of a trumped-up murder rap. Father Daniel Berrigan is set free after serving three years for napalming draft records. Father Philip Berrigan is convicted of smuggling mail out of prison.

I have the best job in the world, writing human-interest feature stories for the *Washington Post*. While the political reporters fuss over the issues of another election year, I get to write about the hopes and disasters of real people. When a Chinese freighter is hijacked by its crew in Baltimore's harbor, I take a speedboat out to drink rice-wine with the mutineers. When a spinster in the Appalachians gets burned out of her house as a witch, I arrive in the sheriff's car, sirens of excitement shrieking in my ears. When a 70-year-old Frenchman beaches his ketch on Assateague Island after sailing the Atlantic alone, I get to Jeep down the surfline to welcome him ashore.

I have just turned 30. I am married to my college girlfriend from our hometown of Detroit. Carol and I are two middle-class kids pretending to be grown-ups. We are good friends, but intimacy has eluded us. We live with our two children in the liberal new town of Reston, Virginia. I am sporting a big Jerry Rubin beard to let my editors, and everybody else, know just where I stand. Yet when I read *The Electric Kool-Aid Acid Test* I am crushed to find out that I have missed the bus. By a mile.

Then the new neighbors move in next door.

It's a Saturday in February. I'm alone downstairs in our modernist townhouse when I see them carrying boxes past on the walkway in front. I should go out and greet them: "Welcome aboard! Want a hand?" Instead, I spy on them through the filmy curtains, trying to make out the shape of things to come.

They're a couple about our age. Like us, they have an older girl and a blond-haired boy. I can't help but notice the wife—what are their names again?—the sleepy, syrupy way she moves, her jeans slung low like a teen-ager.

I hear them carrying stuff up the stairs. Our three-story houses are laid out the same but in reverse. Just a six-inch wall separates our front door, our staircases, our living room, our master bedroom, from theirs.

They sound like Southerners, he kind of twangy, she more silken and slow-drawl.

Linda, that's her name. Long brown hair parted in the middle like Joan Baez. But prettier. Dark-eyed, soft-shouldered, slouchy, tanned. Quilted patches on her ass.

I spy a housewife who wants to be a hippie.

For years I've been arguing with Carol about money. Then we meet the new neighbors, and who cares how many phone calls she makes back to Detroit? The first night that Linda and Rick come over, it doesn't take long for us to slip down off the furniture and sit in a circle on the Rya rug. That's the custom of the day, and usually it serves as a facilitator for passing a joint.

Carol is a loyal beer drinker. She can take pot or leave it. Not me. These days I am drawn helplessly toward couples who smoke. This drug suits my rebel streak, my younger-brother friskiness, my yearning to be different. On the weekends, getting stoned is my No. 1 priority, and I'm hoping Linda and Rick will be game.

Ten minutes into the evening, I bring up the subject.

Linda reaches into the watch pocket of her Levis, and I am dazzled. She's the one who carries their stash.

Immediately we are all best friends. It's one of marijuana's marvels: the openness, the willingness, the trust. We discover that we've been to the same antiwar marches on the Mall. We're all on the McGovern bandwagon. We take turns mocking the system that keeps us afloat. Carol puts on a Carly Simon album. Linda runs next door (I watch her bare feet skipping across the hardwood) to get the Stones. Soon we're all boogieing to *Brown Sugar*.

Wow! She's so playful. So eager to connect. Who wouldn't like her? She has these tender bags under her eyes, little stormclouds of hurt. She has the trace of a mustache on her lip. She is perfumed with patchouli oil, and she's from Savannah. Savannah, Georgia.

She rolls us another joint, expertly. She asks Carol all about her preschool teaching job. She wants to know what it's like to be a reporter for the *Post*. I tell her about being tear-gassed by Nixon's plainclothes thugs when the Yippies took over D.C., and she begs to hear more.

After that night, it's hard for the four of us—well, the two of us—to stay apart. We wait for the weekends to get here. Then we start partying on Wednesdays, then on Thursdays, too, then Tuesdays. We lionize ourselves as pushing the frontiers of evolution, punching holes in the stodgy old workweek, establishing new beachheads against conformity. Is it just a coincidence that our children have also become best friends? We are already joking (at least Linda is) about starting a commune.

Carol is not so enamored. She's uneasy about all the dope smoking. She worries: "What if Andy gets the croup?"

I level: "You get more drunk than I get stoned."

In a larger sense, she's right. I'm not considering the kids' welfare at all. Jenny is 6, Andy is 4. Great children—smart and fun-loving and secure in believing that their parents will hold them close until the end of time. Still, all I can think about is that woman next door.

What a year it is: 1972. The *Joy of Sex* is a runaway best-seller. Couples flock to "open-marriage" workshops to swap partners. "Free-love communes" are springing up in the hills. The Supreme Court rules that unmarried people can buy birth-control devices. J.D. Salinger, aged 53, starts an affair with an 18-year-old student. *Deep Throat* comes out. I have a vasectomy. Good-bye consequence.

Linda lets me know that every morning, after Rick leaves for work, she searches through the *Post* looking for my byline. After that, every story I write becomes an invitation, a proposition, a love letter to her.

What writer doesn't thrive on a little attention? Out on assignment now I find myself filtering my observations through her stony sensibilities. How quickly I can intuit which campy insinuations and off-kilter quotes will make her laugh, which lines in a tear-jerker will showcase my sensitivity. Linda is so easy to please, and my stories have an extra lilt to them now, a poetic liftoff.

One Tuesday in April, on my lunch hour, in Room 628 at the soon-to-be-famous Watergate Hotel, she and I surrender to our greed. We let nature run its majestic course, and it feels so good to be bad that we skip out without paying.

The next day I'm still dizzy from her fragrance when I go to cover the funeral of a boy named Ivan Arnold who died in an orphanage. My sole aim in life now is to make her feel everything I'm feeling. Driving the company Plymouth back to the office, I smoke a big fat one and tune in to her frequency, and the words rain down through the roof:

"Ivan Arnold was here briefly, then gone. An illegitimate child, a foster child, an inward child, an angry child, now no child at all, not a man, but dead..."

Ben Bradlee is charmed and puts it on the front page. In the morning, first thing, I get a call from my No. 1 fan. What a job I've got. They pay me to write these offerings. Then they deliver them right to her doorstep.

My assignments begin to mirror my own explorations. The search to find therapeutic uses for LSD...the family that crosses the ocean in a salvaged ferryboat...the man who gets a sex-change operation. To me, they are singing the same one-note hallelujah, to personal freedom. The freedom to follow your wildest impulses, to do whatever you feel like doing. These stories, while obeying every canon of journalistic objectivity, all end up celebrating my own mutiny against my well-ordered past and my mistress's emancipation and the whole flabbergasting glory of this stopping-point in time.

What a year it is: 1972. Nixon flies off to meet Mao. Muskie cries in New Hampshire. George Wallace gets shot in Maryland. Bobby Fischer beats Boris Spassky in Reykjavik. George Carlin is arrested for reciting The Seven Words You Can Never Say on Television. Clifford Irving admits that he faked the Howard Hughes biography. DNA is conceived. The first hand-held calculator goes on sale. The first compact disc. The first Eagles album. The first Egg McMuffin.

And (how can I forget?) on June 17th of 1972, Nixon's burglars break into the Democratic headquarters at the Watergate. The next day Bob Woodward and Carl Bernstein are hot on the trail. But I am too engrossed in my own Watergate scandal to care about that limp imitation.

To titillate my vamp from Savannah, I slip suggestive words into my stories. One day it's "shaft," the next day "snake," the next day "slippery." When she finds the day's naughty nugget, she calls me at the office. Then she turns the game around. She starts assigning me the words. And even as Bob and Carl keep raising the stakes with Nixon, so that woman keeps raising them with me.

It's a hell of a year for the empowered female: 1972. *Ms.* magazine hits the newsstands. Women run in the Boston Marathon for the first time. The country gets its first female FBI agent, its first female rabbi. Congress passes the Equal Rights Amendment.

It's a year of unraveling: 1972. In his book *A Nation of Strangers*, Vance Packard writes about the decline of the American family and the loss of community ties. From 1970 to 1975, the U.S. divorce rate skyrockets from 33% to 48%.

Once I was such a scrupulous young newspaperman, such a blindly dutiful husband and father. Now I do whatever tickles my sweetmeat's fantasies and write it off to the times. This is a whole new era we're manifesting, of pleasures first and questions later.

Here is my excuse.

When the 1960s broke out, there were lots of young people my age—the war babies, the pre-boomers—who were caught in the middle. The civil-rights and free-speech movements exploded just after I'd finished college and gotten married and started a career and had a child, all by the age of 23. I seemed barely too settled to go south, to join the revolution. But I was way too young to escape its siren song. So over the years I have kept my establishment job and atoned for it by growing a beard, smoking dope and writing indignant memos accusing the *Post* of racism.

If in the '60s I missed out on marching to Montgomery, at least in the '70s I can thumb my nose at Ben Bradlee. If I once lost the chance to tear down my unjust society, at least I can tear apart my unresponsive marriage.

For people who are disaffected but morally ambivalent, marijuana is the perfect drug. It's a poke in the eye to propriety and good order. Yet to enjoy it requires no commitment except, if you choose, to light up again.

It's a year of calamitous deceit: 1972. One by one, the lies are uncovered. Nixon's lies. My lies.

My affair is found out—at 3:30 in the morning, in Linda's living room, by her husband, who'd been listening (for two hours) from the top of the stairs.

I separate from Carol and retreat to a monastic room a block from the *Post*. The decision is all mine. I can do the decent thing and return to my wife and children. Or I can do the delicious thing and surrender myself to Linda's titillations day and night for the next fifty years. Linda is waiting for me to decide, but playing it safe by staying with Rick. Carol is waiting for my answer. Rick is, too. Even the four unknowing children seem to be pleading to know whose daddy I'm going to be, and the ramifications of either decision are unbearable.

I see a shrink once a week. But what really helps is the therapy I do on myself night after night in my room. It consists of filling up the bathtub, climbing in, getting stoned, then lying back in the steaming water to leave my body behind and free-associate about who I am and what I want out of life.

How have I managed to survive into my thirties without once looking at these questions?

In the bathtub (working the faucets with my toes) I understand how wrong it was to blame my workaday father for not being an inspiring figure. He came of age during the Depression and sacrificed any ambitions of his own to provide my brother and me with a stable upbringing in a decent neighborhood. By staying with a job he didn't like, he gave us all that he had to give. For the first time, lying with the water up to my chin, I feel grateful to have had the father I did, and to wish he'd lived past 50.

In the bathtub I understand how fully my character was scripted by my place in the family, as the second born. I see how I steered clear of any fields my big brother Jerry had mastered—carpentry, music, scholarship—because I had no competitive fire. I happily filled the niches that were left for me, as the clown and the athlete. I see how my earliest ambitions were all negative ambitions—to *not* be who my father and brother were, to *not* be serious, to *not* be careful, to *not* be well-behaved—to be anyone but them.

In the bathtub I understand how pitifully unequipped I was to be married at 22. I remember how I expected Carol to leave her parents and sisters behind in Detroit to follow my career to Washington; how

I complained that she was too attached to them, that she should focus on our new family, instead. But I confess to myself now that I was more absorbed in my job than I was in the family.

Over the months, I come to trust those observations and intuitions which appear to me as I lie stoned in the tub. I come to believe that my straight perceptions are too often clouded by intellectual considerations like fear of the unknown or fear of what other people would think. Stoned perceptions seem to well up from deeper within.

Making decisions is a snap now. I just have to look at the question stoned, then act accordingly.

Thus in November, after Nixon wins by a landslide, my own results come pouring in. I conclude that I can live with an Everest of guilt if I have to, but I can't give up this addiction to being so desired, this wonder of being present at the miracle of my stonedmate's transfiguration, this conviction that I am the prince of her awakening.

I ask her to marry me.

Alas, while I've been underwater discovering myself, Linda has been discovering something, too: She needs more of that new currency, that freedom, than one man alone can provide. Our affair has unleashed within her a longing, a confusion, that she cannot contain. All I want is the freedom to be with her, but her need is for freedom itself.

Sure, she will keep reading my newspaper stories and divining their hidden meanings. Yes, she still loves me. But not only me. I'm just being old-fashioned.

It's a year of struggle and carnage: 1972. Vietnam. Bloody Sunday in Ulster. The slaughter at the Munich Olympics. The plane crash in the Andes; the survivors eating the flesh of the dead.

I have one salvation. To get back into the bathtub.

Here, in my cannabinoid trance, I see that Linda is daring me to get angry, to strike back, even to hit her, as some men have. Then she can write me off as just like the others. So I resolve to deny her that satisfaction. It is the only way I can make sense of everything I have won and lost: to set the example for both of us, to keep loving her, but without needing her. As low as I feel, I have to take the high road, in every sense of the word.

I swear off calling her. She will call me, to stay embedded in the war zone of my heart. When she does call, I alternately flirt with her and lavish her with Platonic kindness. I have to be faultless—to make it clear who's to blame for our crash-and-burn. My love is now a curse.

What a year: 1972. At the end of it, Roberta Flack is crooning our farewell—strumming our pain with her fingers, singing our lives with her words, killing us softly.

1973
Getting Brokawed

My marriage is beyond salvation. Carol has a new man, and they're moving to Toronto with our children. Jenny and Andy will visit me in the summers and at Christmas. In the meantime, I am dropping out: quitting the *Post* and moving west. I picture living in Aspen or Sausalito, tending bar, writing novels. This is what Linda and I were going to do: play gypsy together. I can't let her defection stop me.

Then I meet a princess who's heading the same way.

Every Saturday I hitchhike out to Reston to see the kids. Carol and I take the time to catch up, and she keeps mentioning a new friend named Holly who works with her at the preschool. She says this Holly is blond and beautiful and bright and creative. Oh, and beautiful—did she mention that? Carol is such a schemer. Is she playing matchmaker to keep me from ending up with Linda?

Holly is separated from her husband after having an affair. She has two sons. Once she was a debutante. She worked at *Harper's Bazaar*, as the hats and furs editor. But the times are a-changing, and so, I gather, is Holly.

We meet one night at her lakeside home in Reston. Six of us, including an old boyfriend of hers, are sitting in a circle around a candle. We have all taken LSD. Supposedly Holly is planning to move to Aspen at some point to live with this guy. But wait one minute! She and I don't dare to look at each other, for what it would reveal. The flame of the candle wanders this way and that as if pointing a finger each time someone lets out a breath. What's going on? Holly and I have this colossal secret. We cannot let our eyes meet, for what might happen next.

She has on jean short-shorts cut ragged, with a knit top that shows off the curve of her long neck. Her voice is throaty, froggy, original.

When she walks she swings her arms with gusto almost like a man, and I can see the person she's becoming: an outdoorswoman, a Westerner. She is vibrating with the unspent promise of a woman who is just realizing that she can choose her own course in life. She's making the same leap I am making, from remote-control to self-control, and it's breathtaking to behold: a lady like her just bursting into bloom.

This is the first time she has tried LSD. She wants to have it both ways, I can see—to play the good girl, too. Back in school, she tells us, she couldn't enjoy the weekends unless she did her homework first. But this Holly here is a whole other animal. This Holly isn't planning ahead at all. This Holly is ready for whatever comes next.

Unhinged by the acid from earthly limitations, I run over to her open staircase and make an acrobatic flip which leaves me hanging by my ankles and swinging upside-down like an ape, barking some Congolese mating call. I feel a reckless energy racing through my every muscle—a wicked certainty that Holly is aching to let loose, too.

Later we all go skinny-dipping in the lake. After a while, her boyfriend and the others go back into the house. Holly and I are alone, and it's too soon yet for anything to happen. But, as we breast-stroke through the moonlight, her outstretched fingertips barely graze mine, and the shock waves ripple out to touch the farthest shores.

We've got no time to date, to feel each other out. She's moving to Connecticut with her kids for the school year. I've given notice at the *Post*, and I'm getting ready to drive west. Then she asks one simple question:

"Do you want to stop in Connecticut on the way out?"

Is her geography that bad?

Do I care? It's an open-ended invitation.

On the second day of October I drive my Ford Econoline hippie van with the shag-carpeted interior up to Westport, Connecticut. She comes out of her house to greet me in the driveway, and I'm knocked out—DAMN!—by how pretty she is.

A few minutes later, I hang my denims in her closet, and, as easy as that, we're a couple. For how long? For a week? For a month? For a lifetime? We'll take it day by day. What a wonderful time in history this is to be alive.

Oh, yes. I also introduce myself to her two boys, who are 6 and 3, and who asked for none of this.

Holly is a rebel like me. The next summer we carry out our plot to decamp from the material world. We drive out to Colorado, playing *Rocky Mountain High* on the eight-track, to take up the hippie life. We rent a log cabin at elevation 9,000, at road's end, where the snow-plow turns around. We give her kids the only bedroom, so we can sleep by the living-room window looking out upon the snow-laden pines and up at the stars. What a way to start a romance.

In the deep of winter, we have to tunnel through the snow to get to our front door. Drifts sweep up to the eaves. What an adventure it is for a city boy and a suburban girl—learning how to take care of ourselves. I go out into the woods and bully over dead aspens and bust them into firewood. Holly buys cross-country skis for the four of us, and we slip away into the pine forests out back, along the rushing river. When Christmas approaches, we chop down a ponderosa and pull it back on a sled and decorate it with homemade ornaments.

We are like a family, sort of. But the step-dynamics are rugged. The older boy, Scott, is angry. His parents have split. Mom has shanghaied him to dropoutsville. He worships his father, a management consultant in New York. He can't fathom why Mom would throw away the world's all-time greatest human being for a hairy loser like me. His outbursts set the tone in our house, but Holly can't bring herself to discipline him, and I don't have the authority. I don't want it. I am the bemused uncle, likeable enough and possibly reliable, yet untested and probably stoned.

The hamlet we adopt as our mountain home is a historic gold-mining camp dating to the 1850s. After the gold got played out, the town fell into a long decline. A new wave of pioneers arrived in the 1960s, and by the time Holly and I land here it's a hippie heaven on earth. The roads are dirt. The houses are old miners' cabins, some fixed up more than others, most of them tilting a bit. Vegetarians have taken over the General Store and outlawed meat. Our neighbors are playing at being Indians, building sweat lodges in their yards, chanting to the moon, passing a peace pipe in one direction and a dope pipe in the other.

The princess and I jump right in.

With my newspaper career kaput, I take some pleasure—and even pride—in doing menial labor. I land a job down in the city as a janitor in a jewelry store. The owner can't believe he has a *Washington Post* reporter polishing his silver. I drive an ice-cream truck (*ding-a-ling, ding-a-ling*), sneaking tokes between stops, reaching back to grab creamsicles for myself (*ding-a-ling*).

I settle in to painting houses at a new development in Boulder. I spend all day with two other bozos staining window and door casings. When it's break-time, we duck out into the woods to "get stained," as we call it. Then we return to work, and in these moments it is a satisfying occupation, indeed—picking up the brush and dipping the clean bristles into the stain, which is a rich walnut brown, and applying it in long smooth strokes onto the unfinished pine. It's breathtaking to watch the stain sink into the wood and magically bring out the grain.

I dip the brush back into the can, more delicately this time. Then my steady hand and my eagle eye conspire to cut a perfectly clean line where the casing meets the drywall, so there's no work left for the touch-up crew.

I still do some free-lance journalism. So I write a story for the *Post* about industrialized house-building—how the process is broken down into assembly-line jobs like mine. I write that the lack of accountability can lead to errors such as crooked doorways. It's a thoughtful story, harking back to my grandfather, who was a house carpenter.

The day after it's published, a producer for *The Today Show* calls and invites me to come on the program and expand on my revelation about workmen smoking grass on the job. I could tell him that the story is really about construction trends. But marijuana is a hot topic now—its increasing popularity, its perceived risks, the drive to legalize it. Besides, this invitation is a writer's dream come true.

They schedule me for the day after Labor Day, 1977. Tom Brokaw will interview me. I call my widowed mother in Detroit and tell her to tune in. She is pleased to hear it and alerts all of her friends.

NBC puts me up in a hotel near Rockefeller Center. I have rehearsed what I plan to say. Sure, they like the marijuana angle. But I am certain that I can direct Brokaw's attention to the larger issues involved.

Suddenly we are sitting in front of the cameras. Brokaw gives the lead-in. Then he turns to me and says, "So, Tom, in the middle of the morning you and your friends don't take a coffee break, do you? You take a..."

What can I say?

"A marijuana break."

And so it goes. We play fill-in-the-blanks. Brokaw doesn't give me one opening to sing my own song. He even gets me to imply that dope is to blame for the doorways being crooked. He's such a pro at making the point they want to make: that our hippie counterculture is a joke.

I think about my poor mother and her friends, having to see me exposed as a drug addict.

The interview ends. I am ushered off-stage. Willard Scott, the weatherman, who's getting ready to do his next forecast, calls to me across the set: "Hey, Tom! I just bought a condo in Steamboat Springs. You didn't have anything to do with that project, did you?"

The crew has a good laugh. My handler leads me away. Through an open doorway I glimpse a video monitor replaying my appearance. I'm appalled to see how stupid I look, how out of place, in my mountain-man beard and Paul Bunyan get-up. I look glassy-eyed, like I'm stoned.

Do they do that with a special lens?

1977
Situation NORML

After the Brokaw flim-flam, I go to Washington for an assignment that an old *Post* colleague recommended me for. The National Organization for the Reform of Marijuana Laws wants a proposal for a book about cannabis. It's supposed to be a history, a reference work, a how-to, a medicinal guide, a voice for legalization and (as I see it) a lyrical documentation of the lifestyle.

NORML's office is a row house at 2317 M Street NW, between Georgetown and the White House. There I meet its founder, Keith Stroup, and the other young lawyers who are working to loosen the grip of anti-marijuana laws and to provide legal help to growers and users who get busted.

They show me to the third-floor attic room where I'll be sleeping for a few weeks while I research the book. We sit down to pass a joint around, as if to close the deal. At the end, the roach is tossed into a huge glass jar that sits on a table at the head of my bed. The jar looks to be half full of roaches—the last remains, it appears, of hundreds of such business meetings.

They tell me that when NORML helps growers get out of legal troubles, the growers express their gratitude by sending NORML samples of their most outstanding products. So these roaches, which I am invited to consume freely during my tenure, represent a confluence of good will and good weed perhaps unmatched in all of human experience.

The marijuana lobby is on a roll.

Keith Stroup founded NORML in 1970. That was the year Richard Nixon signed the Controlled Substances Act, which listed cannabis for the first time as a Schedule 1 drug—as dangerous as heroin and with no possible medical benefits. Congress named a National Commission on Marijuana and Drug Abuse, and in 1972 it concluded that grass was harmless enough that possession of up to an ounce ought to be legal.

Nixon rejected the report out of hand. Keith Stroup used it to campaign for legal reforms on the state level. During this period, thirty states reduced sentences for possession. When Jimmy Carter ran for president in '76, he came out for decriminalization. The momentum was building.

Now it's 1977. Carter is in the Oval Office. Keith is invited to the White House to have lunch with the president's drug-policy adviser, Peter Bourne, a British-born psychiatrist who once spoke at a NORML conference. Things are getting chummy. NORML's lawyers start playing softball against a team of White House staffers.

That summer, Keith is asked to help draft a big drug speech the president will give to Congress. Carter tones it down, but in August, three weeks before I move into NORML's headquarters, Jimmy delivers the speech, proposing to end all federal penalties for possessing less than an ounce. The editors of the *New York Times* and the fusty *National Review* also come out for decriminalizing.

Meanwhile, Keith is getting high with the Allman Brothers, Jimmy Buffet, Willie Nelson, Hugh Hefner and the president's son Chip. Keith gets sleepovers at the Playboy Mansion. Mr. Marijuana, they call him.

At the time, I am aware of none of this. I'm the ascetic who lives in the attic, smoking the leftovers.

No matter how many of those gift roaches I consume, the jar keeps filling up. Like loaves and fishes.

I make a list of people to interview for the book. Jack Nicholson, Hunter Thompson, Tom Robbins, Dr. Andrew Weil, Peter Lawford,

Sterling Hayden, Lily Tomlin, Tommy Smothers, John Belushi, Geraldo Rivera, Garry Trudeau, the philanthropist Stewart Mott, the tycoon Max Palevsky, and a UPI reporter who boasts of having smoked in a bathroom at the Executive Mansion, and aboard Air Force One, and on Nixon's trip to Peking to meet Mao.

Another promising subject is Fletcher Knebel, a liberal political columnist and the author of the novel *Seven Days in May*. In 1972 he wrote a magazine article describing his first run-in with marijuana at the age of 56, in Mexico: "Warm afternoon sunlight poured over Tepoztlan. Cathedral bells tolled, distant dogs barked, birds skittered through the laurel trees, and by twilight, after only four drags on a joint, I had attained a blissful attitude unknown since first love."

Marijuana, he declared, was "beautifully adapted to people at the tag end of life who get a bit bored with the repetitive rhythms of survival. It has brought me new friends, a rediscovery of music, an awareness of the riches of the senses, a self-knowledge, an inner contentment, and a feeling of excitement seldom felt since I was a child."

On a Friday in September, on the eve of his 66th birthday, I take a train up to see Fletcher Knebel at his home on the wooded outskirts of Princeton, New Jersey. He takes me into his office overlooking the backyard swimming pool. We sit in deck chairs and partake of his Colombian.

"It took me a while," he reflects, "but after two or three years I learned that if I had a problem in my life that I felt was very important to me, and I was torn about it, the best way for me to figure out how I felt...I would come out here to the office, lock the door, and smoke a good strong joint. I'd just sit here and let my mind wander to the problem, and it wouldn't be ten seconds"—he snaps his fingers—"and I'd know precisely how I felt."

One time he got involved in a movie project. He loved the material, but felt uneasy about writing for Hollywood. "So I smoked some grass. And within a minute I realized that it was too complicated for me to figure out why I felt this way, but I did feel that, goddammit, I did not want to do it. So I called and told them, sorry. All I knew was that the grass said: Don't do it. It was such a relief!"

Fletcher Knebel has the munchies. He goes into the kitchen and comes back with a health-food bar.

Dope has liberated him from his inhibitions, he says. He never liked to dance; now he cuts loose. He used to get anxious about having sex; not anymore. He gets away with firing up his pipe in restaurants and on airplanes. One night he saw 500 images of his wife, each one smiling.

He circles back to the subject of old age:

"That's the real time to be smoking it. Because it's not hard for most young people to be fairly flexible, but the longer you live the more deep-set each habit pattern gets. It's almost a standing joke that elderly people are rigid in their ways. And therefore to smoke, say, from age 50 on is just wonderful, to keep you more supple in your attitudes, and thereby enjoy life one helluva lot more."

He thinks the federal government should provide free marijuana to anyone over 50 who has paid his or her taxes. He thinks hospitals should hand it out to their patients.

My cassette tape expires. Have three hours gone by?

Fletcher drives me to the Princeton campus, and we stroll around admiring the architecture and the emerging colors of autumn. We sit down on a slope of emerald grass dappled with fallen leaves and become deeply immersed in a spirited game of tennis. Back and forth... back and forth. The players are young, the volleys are furious. It's late in the afternoon, still golden warm. What a day! Fletcher Knebel marvels at their pinpoint shots.

I return to Colorado in October to write the proposal and resume my adventure with Holly. That same month, Keith Stroup starts coming down from Cloud Nine.

Canadian customs agents bust him for having a joint on him while he's entering the country. At the airport on his way out, they find another joint, plus traces of cocaine. He spends a night in jail and is kicked out of Canada.

Back in Washington, the big issue for NORML is the herbicide paraquat. Since 1975 the federal government has funded a campaign in Mexico to destroy marijuana fields by spraying them with paraquat. Tests indicate that 13% of the pot being smuggled in is tainted with paraquat, and government scientists are warning users that it's unsafe.

Keith persuades Senator Charles Percy to introduce a bill outlawing federal support for the spraying. Keith asks his White House friend Peter Bourne to support the bill. But the administration has been lobbying against it, and Bourne turns him down. Mr. Marijuana is outraged. To him, the government is deliberately poisoning smokers.

To get back at Bourne, Keith leaks a piece of information to syndicated columnist Jack Anderson—about something that happened at NORML's 1977 Christmas party.

It was a great party. A Virginia grower donated a pound of dynamite weed, and volunteers rolled an endless supply of fatties. Some 500 people came, including Capitol Hill staffers and journalists from the straight media. Hunter Thompson was there...Tom Forcade of *High Times* magazine...Hefner's daughter Christy...Bobby Kennedy's son David...Bill Paley, the son of the CBS founder. And Peter Bourne from the White House was there.

What Keith reveals to Jack Anderson later is that Bourne snorted coke at the party, in plain view. (Thompson gasped, "My God, man, we'll all be indicted!")

After the story breaks, Carter's drug policies take on a more sinister look. With his political fortunes sagging, he changes course on decriminalization, and the government starts prosecuting marijuana cases more aggressively. The press chimes in with stories about the dangers of dope.

The movement to legalize runs aground. Two years later Reagan is president, and Nancy launches her Just Say No. The unsavory spread of crack cocaine brings a backlash against all drugs. Keith is replaced at NORML, which is struggling financially and wracked by internal feuds.

During the 1970s, eleven states decriminalized pot; in the '80s, none do. The number of marijuana users in the country is said to drop by 10 million. Public support for legalization, after increasing from 12% to 28% during the '70s, stagnates until the turn of the millennium.

The moment has passed.

So has the time for books about the glories of ganja.

1978
Tossie Turns On

Holly's parents, Chet and Tossie Young, are country-club bigots who live in Bronxville, New York. They didn't approve of her first husband because he was Jewish. Then, after six years, just as they were getting used to the guy, Holly left him. Chet and Tossie hoped their only daughter would come to her senses now and settle down with a proper Anglo-Saxon lawyer or doctor.

Instead, she has chosen me.

What's their problem? My Rutherford B. Hayes beard? My total lack of interest in accumulating money?

Tossie (born as Florence) is the family's aristocrat. Her father, Roy C. Holliss, was president of the New York *Daily News* in the 1940s. Tossie grew up to be a handsome, engaging woman; she modeled for Camel cigarettes. But she had one debilitating passion that ran in the family.

That was for alcohol.

Her father was killed when his car slammed into a tree in Connecticut early one morning in August of 1946.

Seventeen years later, Tossie and Chet's son, Robin, met the same fate.

Robin was Holly's only sibling. He was two years older than she was, the one more likely to get in trouble. When Holly was 19 and going to Bennett College an hour and a half north of Bronxville, she and her roommate Sheila set up a double-date. Robin would be Sheila's date. He drove up from Bronxville with Holly's date, and they all partied.

Driving home, the boys wiped out. Robin was found in the driver's seat, barely alive. He spent two days in a coma before he died. Chet and Tossie couldn't talk about it with Holly. Holly couldn't talk about it. She still can't. She has virtually never brought it up with me.

I will also go on to lose my only brother, and I'll feel the need to tell people all about it. Invariably I'll get choked up. But Holly's grief—and maybe her guilt—seem to be buried with Robin.

She herself hasn't inherited the drinking gene. I'd expect her to be either very susceptible or very averse to alcohol. Instead, she will nurse one glass of wine, or two at a party. She is a woman who keeps herself under control at all times. Nobody will ever catch Holly Young stumbling around or slurring her words.

She is just as moderate with marijuana. She enjoys it socially. We use it to jack up the mood for lovemaking. But I've never known her to light up by herself. She gets stoned when she's invited, but she isn't a stoner.

When Holly was growing up, her mother quit drinking. But ever since then, it seems, Tossie hasn't found another way to get light-hearted and carefree. As fate would have it, their whole crowd is a happy-hour crew, and Chet is the life of the party. In Bronxville, and after they retire to Florida, they spend most of their evenings at cocktail parties, where Tossie resents Chet for always having to be the center of attention.

The Tossie that I know can be witty and occasionally hilarious. But too often she seems cranky and bedeviled by health problems which baffle every doctor money can buy.

Also, she plainly has no use for me. When Holly goes down to Florida to visit them every spring, Tossie keeps inviting the same eligible bachelor over for happy hour.

By the holiday season of 1977-'78, Holly and I have been living together for four years. Chet and Tossie must figure they're stuck with me, because they invite us both to spend a few days with them at a resort in Puerto Rico.

Naturally, I take some weed with me, along with a little LSD. Why shouldn't I see Puerto Rico at its most astonishing? Plus, Holly wants her mother to try smoking grass. She has been on a campaign to help Tossie find some way, any way, to enjoy her later years. She has urged her to take up meditation. Recently Holly asked her about marijuana, and Tossie showed some flicker of interest.

Our first day in Puerto Rico is my 36th birthday. Holly and I borrow Chet's rental car and drive to the El Junque rain forest and drop acid. We get away from the trails and take off our clothes and swim under waterfalls and swing on jungle vines like Tarzan and Jane. Later we drive to the beach and lie down side by side in the sandy shallows and let the surf roll us up and down like logs.

That night we're going to eat out at the resort's restaurant—Holly and me, her parents and Tossie's sister Anne, another reformed drinker who also might want a toke.

First, we have cocktails in our condo. Chet mixes gin-and-tonics for the willing. Tossie and Aunt Anne start slugging down Shirley Temples. Then Holly brings it up: "Mom, would you like to try that thing we talked about?"

Tossie pretends to be annoyed. "Oh, I suppose so."

I wonder if Chet might object. Instead, he's amused to see me reach into my shirt pocket and pull out a joint.

I demonstrate its proper use, then hand it to Holly. She takes a suck and makes a point of holding the smoke in.

Tossie tries it, her face scrunched up in self-dismay. She exhales, but nothing comes out.

"I don't how to do this," she complains.

Chet laughs.

Holly coaxes, "Try it again, Mom."

She does, with a visibly better result.

Chester Young is an old New York advertising man. He has seen a lot in his time. But this is the craziest thing he has ever witnessed—his wife Tossie smoking marijuana. He goes over to the bar and pours himself another G & T.

The conversation gets more tentative. We're waiting for something to happen.

Finally Tossie announces, "Well, I don't feel anything at all!" She acts cheated. "It doesn't work for me!"

She asks her sister. "Does it work for you?"

Aunt Anne shakes her head no.

Tossie turns to Holly. "I knew it wouldn't work."

Chet looks pleased, even ennobled, by the outcome.

A short time later, we're heading out the door, going to dinner. Tossie steps into the heat of the tropical night. Suddenly she pulls up short and looks around, in every direction. She gazes up into the treetops. Her face is a mask of utter amazement.

"MY LORD!" she exclaims. "LISTEN TO THOSE BIRDS!"

Not long after we get back to Colorado, Tossie phones Holly. They chat for a while. Then Mom comes around to it. She's embarrassed to say it: "Do you think Tom could send me a couple more of those..." The word sticks in her throat. She isn't really asking her daughter this, is she? "...a few more of those *joints*?"

I roll up four of them and include a note about which end to light. I mail them off to Ponte Vedra Beach.

How cool is this? I'm Tossie's drug dealer now.

In subsequent phone calls, Tossie says the joints are working. She keeps them in a drawer of her dressing table. In the evenings, while she puts on her makeup before they go out, she takes a puff, then stubs the joint out in her Limoges ashtray. She doesn't do it in front of Chet. He has his own bedroom. He doesn't need to know everything.

Now Tossie has a better time at cocktail parties. Part of the fun is having her little secret. She wonders if people notice that she's more chatty than she used to be, and sometimes downright silly.

She calls Holly every few weeks to ask if I can send another care package. I never thought it would be so easy to worm my way into Tossie's heart. I wouldn't ask her to pay, even if money is the one thing she has that I don't.

Then one day she reads an article in *Reader's Digest* which claims that marijuana is as addictive as alcohol.

Poor Tossie. She never places another order.

1980
My Brother's Killer

In January my brother Jerry disappears on a business trip to San Francisco. His rental car is found along a freeway with a bashed-in front fender, 400 unexplained miles on the odometer, and blood on the front seat.

My mother calls from Detroit with the news, and the next morning I hitchhike down to Denver and get on a bus. I should fly to Detroit; my mom needs me. But I want some time to digest what is happening, to sit looking out the window of an overland bus, to be shipped across the country without a tag, to escape the weight of this new reality for, what, thirty-six hours?

I ride with Trailways instead of Greyhound because they stick to the old U.S. highways, passing houses and farms and crossroads cafes and whole communities where I can see people going on with their lives as if nothing had happened. When we ease through towns in the evening I look into people's windows and see yellow cones of lamplight on the walls and imagine some warmth going on in there.

North Platte. Grand Island. Lincoln. When the bus stops for a rest break I walk around to see what kinds of homes the people have, what kinds of department stores and dimestores and street signs, what kinds of banks and bakeries and water towers and brands of gasoline. Council Bluffs. Des Moines. I have a window seat with room to stretch out, no one beside me. Cedar Rapids. Davenport.

Every couple of hours I slip back into the bathroom and puff on a joint, to open my eyes to new angles, new formulations, new panoramas. Then I go back to gazing out the window and turning over in my mind: What might have happened to Jerry except that one thing we can't accept?

Mom's hope is that he was hit on the head and is wandering around somewhere with amnesia. My hope is that he staged the disappearance in order to ditch his corporate job and his controlling wife—and even his three kids, if that's what it took.

Jerry was always the quiet one, the cautious one. I was the rambunctious one, the careless one. During that night on the bus rolling through Iowa, I have a dream that I'm hitchhiking across the country like I used to do, and a car approaches. I look, and it's Jerry behind the wheel. He's alive! But he doesn't stop for me. He doesn't recognize me. He passes me right by.

When I wake up in the morning we're moving through Illinois, the tires humming their lost-in-time lullaby. I duck into the bathroom... blow the smoke out the miniature sliding window. Then I sit back down and close my eyes and imagine going out to California and playing detective: looking for my runaway brother. I picture finding him roller-skating along a boardwalk with a girlfriend in some beach town south of L.A. I see Jerry and me walking arm-in-arm, acting like buddies for the first time ever.

Still, I keep coming back to what the sergeant told me over the phone, what I won't be telling Mom, about how much blood they found in the car, and how it matched Jerry's type. I wonder about those 400 miles: who drove them and where he went and whether Jerry was along for the ride.

I am haunted, especially, by the sorry truth that I haven't seen my only brother in eight years—since I ran off to Colorado. His wife Liz has written me off as a bad influence: deserting my family, smoking marijuana. She hasn't let Jerry get near me. When he and I talked on the phone on Christmas Day, I told him I wanted to come and see him. Now I can't accept that I've lost my chance.

In Chicago I change buses, and we roll on through the dreary flatlands of Indiana and Ohio as I slowly reconcile myself to the idea that my days as the irresponsible younger brother, the husband who'd leave his wife and kids, the son who'd let his grieving mother sit alone while he road-tripped across America—those days are over. The '70s are over. I am getting ready to be the only child.

The next Sunday night, Mom and I receive the phone call we've been dreading and yet waiting for. Jerry's body was found in a farmer's field in Paso Robles, 200 miles south of San Francisco, with a bullet in his head.

The man who did it, an escaped murderer from Arkansas, has been caught in Arizona after killing more people there. But we don't care about that. We aren't the kind of people who'd ever stand up in a courtroom and cry out for revenge. Instead, we know how to take our medicine. That is Mom's brand of Midwestern strength, and my strength, too.

I hang up the kitchen phone and walk back to her bedroom, the longest walk of my life. She is sitting on the edge of the bed, weeping softly. I sit next to her and put my arm around her, and I cry with her. I cry for her.

I try to let her know how sorry I am. I tell her, "You'll always have me, Mom."

She turns to me, her face all awash. "Please don't let anything happen to you, honey," she whimpers.

I pledge, "I won't, Mom. I promise."

From now on, this will be my assignment.

We fly to Minneapolis for the funeral. I am dazed to finally be in Jerry's house, but without Jerry. I hardly know his teen-aged kids, a girl and two younger brothers. Liz and I hug, but without affection. She had been with Jerry since high school—a short, self-satisfied woman who could dominate a conversation and, I saw, a husband, too.

The funeral is held at Liz's Christian Science church. Beforehand,

I slip out into the alley to smoke a jay, so that I'll be super-aware. I don't want to miss a thing. The service begins, and I'm incensed when the minister mispronounces our last name. I want to jump up and shout, "HOW DARE YOU DISGRACE JERRY! YOU DIDN'T EVEN KNOW HIM!"

But I keep my peace. I didn't know Jerry, either.

That afternoon I put Mom on a plane back to Detroit. Liz drives me to the Trailways station, and we make empty promises to stay in touch. Then I board the bus for Sioux Falls and settle into a window seat.

Now we will begin trying to forget.

Except for me. I want to know more.

The bus rolls into the night, through the frozen stage sets of St. Peter and Mankato. I do that sneaky thing I do in the bathroom. Then I put together what we know. The 200 miles from San Francisco to Paso Robles accounted for the extra 400 on the odometer. The killer kidnapped Jerry and headed south. Later, for some reason, he turned around and drove back up to the Bay Area, where the car was found.

Jerry was shot in the left temple. The blood was all around the passenger seat. So that was where it happened, it seemed. If the killer shot him right away, would he have driven all the way to Paso Robles with the body next to him? No, that didn't make sense. No, Jerry had to be alive for that ride. The two of them must have spent the whole evening sitting side by side in that rental car staring out the window at the onrushing night.

Dope affects us in different ways. It can momentarily embolden a shy person to turn effusive. It can strike a blabbermouth dumb for a while. It puts some of us to sleep and wakes some of us up. But I don't think it changes who you are. It amplifies who you are. It intensifies what you experience and feel. It brings out whatever's inside.

If you have fear, it can make you paranoid. If you are an optimist, it can make you a Pollyanna. If you're a nosy newsie like me who is always curious to know what's up and who loves to tell everybody all about it—then dope will just make you curiouser. And curiouser.

No one else wants to know what happened that night on the highways of central California. My mom's only defense is to put it behind her, as she did when Dad died. Liz is protecting her kids from any more harm. We don't know the fate of the man who killed Jerry. We don't even know the guy's name. But as time goes by—one year, two years, three years—I keep trying to picture that night.

I imagine that Jerry was an obedient hostage. Maybe he was tied up; maybe he didn't have to be. But was he afraid? Did he have to plead for his life? What did they do along the way, the two of them? What did they talk about? Did they have to stop for gas? Did Jerry ever try to get away? Did anything good at all come out of it? Don't we need to get to the bottom of this? Won't the truth, only the truth, give us some final satisfaction?

I get an assignment from *California Magazine* and fly out there to investigate. I pore over the police reports, bewitched: how Jerry was last seen leaving work at 6 p.m.; how at three minutes after midnight two men using Jerry's credit card checked into the Black Oak Motor Lodge in Paso Robles; how Jerry's body was found three miles from the motel; how seven other travelers were murdered by this same man. And, finally, he has a name: Donald Eugene Harding.

In my own rental car, I retrace the route he and Jerry would have taken south out of San Francisco, past freight yards and warehouses and shipping terminals. I leave the city behind, and the pop rock on the radio soon gives way to country tunes. I take a good hit on my traveling pipe.

Past the shapely ghosts of eucalyptus trees.

Past cherry stands closed for the season.

Down the Salinas Valley they drove.

Hurtling through the dark, all that Jerry could have seen was the patch of highway transfixed by the headlight glare, and the glimmer of the instrument panel, and the dim features of the desperado sitting next to him.

Maybe he told Donald Harding something about his life. Maybe they began using each other's first names. Maybe Jerry was confident that he was going to survive this. Maybe he could even see it as exciting, to be seized away from all that he knew to be familiar and correct.

It is 203 miles from the Bay Bridge Holiday Inn, where Jerry was kidnapped, to Paso Robles. It took them five and a half hours. So they must have made some stops.

I find the Black Oak Motor Lodge, in the tourist zone along the 101 freeway at the north end of town. I pull in, and for the first time on the trip I feel uncomfortable. This doesn't feel like a good place for me to be.

It's a two-story Best Western with a pool and well-trimmed shrubbery, a motel Jerry might have chosen. Their room, #209, is on the ground floor. A maid lets me in. But what is there to see? Two double beds. A Gideon Bible. Two Impressionist prints of the same country lane.

Gladly, I get back into the car. Now there is only one more place I have to go—to that farmer's field where Jerry's body was found with his sport coat draped over him.

I head south on the 101, slowly, for one mile, for two miles, following the directions in the police reports.

Was this where he shot him?

Three miles. Was this the place, right here?

I take the exit for Highway 46 West. I turn right at the stop sign, as instructed, then right again along the frontage road, for two-tenths of a mile. I come to a farmed hillside sloping up to a house. I park under a big oak tree at the corner of the property.

I duck through the barbed-wire fence into the field, and I step off twelve feet.

Okay. Here we are.

I once heard Ram Dass say that when a person dies suddenly his spirit can linger around that place on earth, confused about where to go next. So I turn my back to the highway, and I close my eyes. I try to concentrate. I try to relax. But standing here I cannot pick up any feeling for my brother's soul adrift here in time.

And I still can't answer the one question that brought me out to California: How did Jerry spend his final hours? What happened between 6 o'clock that evening, when he left work, and 9:45 the next morning—almost sixteen hours later—when Harding abandoned the car in the East Bay.

I walk into the Fremont Police Department to see the lead detective on the case, Sgt. Bob Pile. He tells me:

"Nobody is going to be able to answer those questions for you. There's only one person in the world who could ever tell you, and that's Donald Harding."

My brother's killer is on Death Row at the Arizona State Prison. When I get back to Colorado, I write him a letter. I tell him that I feel no animosity toward him, and it's true. Then I explain what I'm looking for.

Six days later, when I open our mailbox at the bottom of the driveway, I find an envelope with a remarkable return address and a bulky object inside.

It's unsettling to hold it in my grasp, to picture him sitting in his cell licking these very stamps.

His handwriting is practiced and precise: small block letters of equal height and spacing.

DONALD E. HARDING

P.O. BOX B-43255

FLORENCE, AZ 85232

It reminds me of my father's fine lettering in our family photo albums. Here is one thing, his penmanship, that Donald Harding cares about.

I stand by the mailbox fingering the envelope. What is wrong with me, that I want to recognize his humanity, that I actually relish doing it?

Harding has my address now. I've been imagining what would happen if he broke out of prison, as he has a knack for doing. We're only a day's drive from Arizona. We live in the mountains, a good place to hide. He'd see me as sympathetic. He'd think: Those Huth boys are easy pickins.

I don't want Holly or the kids to see the envelope. This is dirty business. I stop in the driveway and peel it open, careful to preserve the handwriting.

Inside is a cassette tape labeled, in the same neat jailhouse lettering: 8/1/84   APPROX. 45 MINUTES DISCUSSION.

I wait until that night after dinner. Then I put the cassette in my pocket and, with daylight still holding up the western sky, I walk through our recycled ghost town, past the closed-up hotel and the log saloon, past the General Store and the volleyball court and the volunteer firemen's barn, to my writing cabin in the far meadow.

I stand on the old plank porch and pee into the weeds below. I linger here to collect myself, to appreciate the keenness of this moment. I commune with my pipe, because I don't want to miss a thing. I watch the sun's last rays lighting up the ridge above our house. I hear a horse snuffling in a neighbor's corral. Now stillness again.

I go inside and put new batteries into my cassette player. I sit in the chair next to the woodstove.

I slip in the tape, Side A, and press PLAY.

At first, just background noises. A clanking. A scraping noise. Two men shouting at each other.

"TWELVE-THIRTY!"

"WHAT?"

"TWELVE-THIRTY!"

"ON YOUR FEET!"

"WHAT?"

"ON YOUR FEET!"

The shouting subsides. I listen to the uneven grain of the tape.

Then a voice speaks out—so clearly, so intimately, he could be sitting right next to me:

"Tom? Donald Harding here."

First he tells me his own wretched story—how he was sent to a reform school in Arkansas at the age of 10 for running away from home, then sent to the state penitentiary at 15 for running away from reform school. Put simply: "I have been in confinement all of my life, Tom." When he has escaped, he has had no other vision of what to do than to imprison other people—to kidnap them and tie them up and rob them and, if they try anything, to kill them. He can do unto others only as others have done onto him.

I had expected to hear a cockiness in his voice, a foul mouth, an attitude. Instead, he sounds contrite and even sensitive. Here is a man resigned to purgatory. As I sit listening to his tale, I can't feel any malice. I feel sorry for him. At least Jerry had thirty-nine pretty good years. This guy hasn't had a one, and now he's headed for the gas chamber.

The tape plays on, and at last Donald Harding ("Don," he wants me to call him) tells me what happened that night in 1980—how he waylaid Jerry in the Holiday Inn parking lot...how robbery was his only motive...how they stopped two or three times at coffee shops so Jerry could cash travelers checks...how they talked as they drove, about their lives and their beliefs and their lack of religious convictions... how Jerry showed him family pictures. This is such welcome news. It is just what I wanted to hear.

Then he gets to the part where they checked into the Black Oak

Motor Lodge.

I lean forward, to catch his every word.

"When we got to the motel, I rented a room to leave him there—to tie him up and pretend to leave, to see if he could get away, because I had had experiences where I tied people up and they got loose and called the police on me, and I made some narrow getaways. So I tied him up with bedsheets and pretended to leave."

I picture him hiding in the bushes, peering in the window, playing cat and mouse. For him to be free, Jerry had to be in captivity. That was his grim calculation. It had to be one of them or the other.

"And Jerry got out of his, umm...he loosened the knots and was freeing himself of his bonds, I could see. So I went back in the room and told him that I was going to have to take him somewhere else—in the woods somewhere. I was going to try to locate some woods and tie him to a tree. And I didn't want to do it, but I told him, 'You're going to have to rough it out there.' And your brother told me, he said, 'Look...' This was after I had finished untying his hands from the bed. He said, 'Look, leave me here.'

"I said, 'I cannot leave you here, because then I will be captured or killed.' I didn't want to leave him out in the woods. I knew it would be miserable as hell, but that was the alternative I could see. And he told me before we left the room, he said, 'If you're going to kill me, shoot me between the eyes.' He was becoming very apprehensive, and I tried to convince him that I was not going to harm him. But he got para...he just didn't trust the situation.

"And we got back out on the expressway. And, uhhh, well, I had told him at some point during our discussion that I had, you know, that I had, uhhhhhhh, that I had killed people, because it was a necessity."

Symphony music wells up behind him.

"We were driving down the freeway, and I was looking for some isolated woods, and, uh, your brother, uhhh, he kicked me. I nearly wrecked the car. The car skidded, it swerved, and, uhhhh, I shot him.

"It was an impulsive reaction, and he didn't know what hit him. So in saying that I guess I tell you that your brother died bravely in trying to escape. He never at any point cowered, you know."

Silently, I thank him for telling us that.

He says, "I know it sounds so senseless and bizarre, Tom, but that's how it happened. I guess he was trying to make me wreck, and I don't know what he could accomplish. His hands were still tied. He apparently thought that I was going to take him out and kill him. But that wasn't my intention. I tell you this in all sincerity."

Some licks of Southern rock.

"That's the truth of the matter. And again I want to say, Tom, I am very sorry. I'm sorry from the bottom of my heart, that I took your brother's life, probably at a point where he was in the prime of his life. I'm sorry for the grief that it's caused you, and your family and his family, his wife, his children. I'm very sorry."

The radio behind him croons: *"I've cried so hard..."*

"Okay, Tom. Take care. Bye."

I give my mother the choice. I telephone her and say: "I found out how Jerry died, and it wasn't as bad as we might have thought." I offer to send her the magazine story. She replies, evenly, "No, thanks, honey."

I ask if she'd mind relaying the offer to my sister-in-law Liz. A week later Mom tells me Liz is "mortified" that I would even suggest such a thing.

I'm perplexed. If they don't know what happened, won't their minds keep coming up with new scenarios? How will they ever be able to let it go?

*One Adventure
Too Many*

1984
Mountain Mama

After living together for ten years as girlfriend and boyfriend in a motley accrual of rental cabins, Holly and I are making commitments. We get married in a mountain meadow near the village we call home. We look for a house to buy, or for land where we can build.

One deal looks promising—until the owner calls to say that it's off. When I hang up the phone, that old instinct kicks in: to get high and see where it leads. In turn, I wander outside and, following some vague inclination, hike up the hillside above our house. Partway up the ridge sit two log cabins owned by summer people who rarely use them. Both have knockout views of the Continental Divide. One of them has a cabin with two bedrooms standing off by itself. Next to it is a shelf in the hillside where, it seems, an adjoining living space could be built.

I stand on the shelf looking out at the peaks, taking a few sidesteps one way, then the other way, until the vista is perfectly framed by the pines. Okay: This is where I'd put the living room. Big windows. French doors leading out to a deck. Behind me, the kitchen. Upstairs in a loft, our bedroom, with the best view of all.

What makes me think I can build a house? It's so against the grain of my upbringing.

My father, the carpenter's son, had a workbench in the basement. Before I could even walk, I heard Jerry down there happily banging away with him. Later, at elementary school in Detroit, Jerry was the star pupil in shop class. The teacher, Ira Madden, was to industrial-arts education what Betty Crocker was to layer cakes. His best laddies kept winning nationwide woodworking competitions, and Jerry was one of them.

He turned out napkin-holders and letter-openers and other endearing objects for the house. Then he graduated to making wooden serving trays whose intricate geometric designs he rendered in three-dimension by carving out thousands of tiny triangular chips with a razor blade. It was something which must have taken (I could only guess) a cross-eyed amount of focus, dedication and patience.

Did I one-up Jerry by chip-carving us a new front door? No, I rigorously avoided the workbench in favor of that corner of the basement where the pool table squatted.

Still, I had to take shop class. I remember the day Mr. Madden showed off Jerry's latest tray, to inspire us. He looked around to find my chubby face in back. "Tommy!" he hailed. "Why can't you do good work like this?"

I shrugged. "I don't know." My friends snickered.

My strategy was to not try. I spent every class sanding pieces of scrap wood down to nothing while I played sports-trivia games with my pals.

Genius at work: If I didn't try, how could I fail?

Holly is the one who pushed to get married. She's the one who's most eager to have a house of our own. If we build, you can bet that she'll be one of the carpenters.

For a country-club girl, she has proved to be one tough mountain mama. She has refashioned herself into a hiker, a backpacker, a river runner, an off-roads biker. For a debutante who was raised to be merely attractive, she has shown that she has brains too—as a preschool teacher and director, as a poet, as an author.

She is perpetually busy—not ambitious to gain worldly fame, but driven to lead a life of meaning. Even in her hippiest years, the days weren't long enough for everything she wanted to do. She starts each morning with her regimen of meditation and yoga and an exercise walk. Then she has phone calls to make—to thank a friend for a nice evening; to set up a schedule for reading to inner-city kids; to make a date with the teen-aged girl she counsels for a friend-of-the-court program; to make hair or doctors' appointments. Before turning to her writing, she might pen a note in Spanish to the child we sponsor in Guatemala.

My life is way easier. Mainly I sit at my typewriter and get high and think up words. I don't envy Holly for feeling that her work is never finished. She doesn't envy me for doing so little, for being so detached. I feel superior to have a mind uncluttered by distraction and obligation. She feels superior for being on a path to God.

Sometimes she says she wishes I were "more spiritual."

I counter with something innocuous like, "Maybe my spirit shows up in ways you don't notice."

Her desire to lead a meaningful life has made her the model of the new independent woman. She is out to fulfill herself. She has zero interest in doing a man's laundry or fussing over his insecurities. She is someone, it seems, who will always make do for herself—the kind of modern woman who will never need to be taken care of.

I love designing our house on the ridge. I'm the chief architect while Holly is the decorator. We'll have a big window seat up front to gather in the view. We'll have an adobe greenhouse to soak up the Colorado sunshine. I've got just one question: How do you build a house?

We hire an unlicensed contractor, Ed, whose kids go to Holly's school. Holly and I sign on as his crew. My son Andy, 17, flies out from Toronto. Holly's boys pitch in.

Self-sufficiency is the cornerstone of the dropout creed. It feels only natural to build our own house. But it's unreal, too. After all this time—Mr. Madden dead for thirty years...my father dead for twenty-two...my brother gone now, too—I'm coming out of the closet as a carpenter.

A concrete crew pours the slab, 25 feet to a side. Three days later we have the 2-by-6 front wall framed, and what a powerful moment it is, to stand the wall up, then to step back to see how each window captures its own view.

In a neighbor's field we find old timbers to use as the roof beams. At salvage yards we find odd-sized windows and jigsaw them together to make up the greenhouse walls.

By midsummer we're running the wiring and plumbing through the studs. We're stuffing in the insulation. Now, with our builder Ed teaching us every step of the way, we're putting up drywall. We lay out each piece with a massive T-square and cut it with a utility knife. We have to nail it to the studs without cratering the surface. With five novices on the job, there's a continual chorus:

"Hey, Ed...?"

"Hey, Ed...?"

We have to tape the edges. We have to mud between the cracks. We have to sand every surface.

Through face masks now, the chorus muffled:

"Hey, Ed...?"

By August we're trimming out the windows and doors. Painting and staining. A crew comes in to drill a water well 460 feet deep. We anchor a deck to the ponderosas to make the whole place feel like a treehouse.

What a lasting piece of joinery this has turned out to be for our cobbled-together family.

Here in the '80s, as we're affirming our commitments to each other, Holly and I are also making the best friends we will ever have—neighbors, parents like us, couples our age who like to explore the natural world and get high around the campfire rather than working all the time.

This is also the period (drum-roll) when Holly's sons move to New

York to live with their father.

In New York they'll have prep-school educations, big-city stimulation and better sports opportunities. Holly argues for what kids can learn in the mountains: community, nature, stillness. But it's been in the cards all along. The older one, Scott, jumps ship at 13. Two years later he flies out to visit us—a bounty hunter coming to claim his man. When he leaves, he takes Robb with him.

The day that they fly away, I figure Holly will be inconsolable. So that evening I'm dumbfounded when she appears dolled up in a nightie she must have picked up on the way home from the airport at Frederick's of Hollywood.

Do I not understand the first thing about this woman?

The love-in lasts all weekend. She chatters about the book she wants to rewrite, about the time she'll have for her friends, about the walks she'll take with her muse.

Then on Monday she crashes. The whole day goes wrong, and that evening she murmurs as we sit watching the sunset: "I feel empty. Like an empty hole."

"You'll see them at Christmas," I cheer, never at a loss for the obvious.

"He's so young!" she protests. "It's so early!"

"He'll come out next summer."

"It's like one limb is suddenly missing, and I have to learn to walk all over again."

Over the years, I have come to appreciate Scott and Robb. I'm still more of an uncle to them than a father, but that's all we wanted from each other. Now that they're gone, of course, I'm in heaven, having the princess to myself. And it comes with a bonus. We have more freedom to roam. We have learned that we're travelers at heart, and now we don't have a school schedule to tie us down.

In a smoke-induced state of clarity, we decide to break up the long mountain winters by becoming early-onset snowbirds. We buy a midget travel trailer for $850, and every January we tow it to California. For $12 a night we live at state-park campgrounds on the beach. San Clemente. Malibu. Santa Barbara. Every morning we wake up to the cannonading of the surf. Every night we sit around hobo campfires made out of scrap lumber from construction sites.

Beach bums. For fifteen winters straight.

She could have done so much better.

Holly's relationship with her sons changes once they move away.

When they lived with us, she was a good mother, but casual about it, not possessive. When Robb became a hot-shot BMX bike racer, we usually let other parents drive him to the track so we'd have those Sundays alone by ourselves. As soon as the boys leave, though, she longs to hold onto them. From now on she will cherish them, glorify them, do whatever she can to keep bringing them back for more.

In the winters she sets up gala ski trips to Aspen. In the summers she arranges spectacular river trips through the red-rock canyons of Utah. And I love these adventures as much as anyone. The only downside, for me, is that all of our focus as a stepfamily is on vacations aimed at delighting her two jocks rather than my kids.

As a parent, Holly is way more driven than I am. I'm up against one awesome force: the needs of a mother who is awakened by loss. I feel steamrollered by her fixation with pleasing Scott and Robb. I'm flat-out jealous. When her sons are around, I'm invisible to her. It's a bummer that even dope can't dispel.

Later in life I will blame myself for not standing up more forcefully for my children's prerogatives. At the time, it's just easier to let Holly call the shots.

1993
The Beach Shack

I know that some people in the straight world—nurses, doctors, lawyers, bankers, teachers, cops—are secret off-duty stoners who can reconcile the two behaviors and remain part of the system. I have a different outlook. Granted, I hang with a maverick crowd. But I regard habitual, dedicated smokers as individuals who steer clear of social regimentation and authority and who create lives which are idiosyncratic and spontaneous, lives geared more toward valuable experiences than financial security.

In my case, I was contented (hell, I was overjoyed) to be a salaried newspaperman—until I became a pothead. Then I started courting daydreams about becoming a real writer, a writer with a capital W, with no one else to answer to. And it might have happened without the agency of marijuana. But at least marijuana fueled the fire within.

In Colorado in the late '70s I tried writing fiction. I had two novels published, stony satires of the hippie culture. Then I fell into free-lancing feature stories for the big travel magazines.

Traveling, especially to somewhere new, has some of the same tonic effects as smoking weed. It blows open your senses to fresh landscapes of place and time. So it makes perfect sense: Traveling stoned doubles the pleasure.

Other correspondents are sent off to wine and dine in London and Tuscany and Florence. Lucky me, I get Papua New Guinea, the Solomon Islands, Madagascar, Mauritius, Minsk, Murmansk, Tuvalu, Tobago, Bolivia, Honduras, the headwaters of the Ganges, Arctic Finland when it's 30 below, Romania when communism falls, the Andaman Islands to catch glimpses of an uncontacted tribe.

Holly comes along on the trips that interest her. *Outside Magazine* has her do the photos. She's a superb traveler: hardy, enthusiastic, tireless, handy with other languages, unruffled by danger or hardship.

In 1993, we do a month of volunteer work in a village on Lake Atitlan in Guatemala. Then we go next door to sample Belize. On the trip's last morning, we are walking the beach hand-in-hand in a warm rain in a levitated state of consciousness when she fancies: "What if we had a place like this that we could come back to whenever we wanted?"

"A beach house?"

"Not a house, exactly."

"A beach *shack*?" That's more our style.

"With fruit trees in the yard..."

Instantly I grasp the journalistic potential.

"Mangoes," she imagines. "Pineapples. Fresh papayas for breakfast right off the trees..."

"I'd make the railings out of driftwood."

My editors will love it: The beach shack in paradise. Who hasn't dreamt it? You could build it out of thatch or bamboo or adobe bricks or polished hardwoods. You could build it without walls, open to the jungle, like the expats do in Yelapa—bougainvillea crawling over the showerhead. But you'd want to keep it simple, so you'd have less to lose if the local situation turned against you.

Both of us picture a cottage made of 2x4s and planking in the Caribbean style, with brightly painted shutters thrown open to the sea and a tin roof so we could lie in bed listening to the rain. We spent one winter living in a place like that at the farthest end of the last island in the West Indies. With native carpenters I could build it in a month or two, couldn't I? That's how it looks walking blissed out in the rain. We wouldn't need R-19 insulation and double-glazed windows. Wouldn't have to bury our pipes six feet under. Wouldn't need windowglass at all.

It must have something to do with turning 50. I am shadowed by the fact that one month after my father reached 50 he toppled off a couch in Saginaw, Michigan, with a heart attack and died before he hit the floor. Holly and I are still healthy and active and fit. But it's not crazy to wonder how many more adventures we have left in us.

I land an assignment from Conde Nast *Traveler* to scout out a homesite in Costa Rica, which is emerging as a trendy destination. The next winter, the two of us drive down its Pacific coast for six weeks, exploring the possibilities. We don't find anything that suits our funky tastes or our budget until we come to the untouristed shores of the Golfo Dulce (the Sweet Gulf), down near the Panama border.

The Armpit of Costa Rica, gringos call it—hot, humid, rainy, buggy, lawless. The squatters wear sidearms. I've saved this coast for last.

The town of Golfito is a spent-out banana-belt port that was abandoned by United Fruit after labor troubles in the 1980s. From here it's a four-hour drive on primitive roads and across jerrybuilt bridges to the end-of-the-line peninsula of Zancudo. Which is Spanish for mosquito.

Small cottages hide back among the coconut palms and almond trees. The beach is broad and flat and fringed with driftwood. The waves look ideal for body-surfing.

We meet other gringos who are building—the teachers from Mendocino, the woodworker from Aspen, the gold-miners from Dawson City, the letter-carrier from Quebec. We pick up an aura of shared romance like the one we found in Colorado in the 1970s, that sense of being on a frontier together, but an agreed-upon frontier, already staked out.

With some of Holly's inheritance, we buy 250 feet of beachfront. My editors turn it into a three-part series. *The Eden Project*, they call it. We return to build the shack, and Annie Leibovitz flies down to photograph us.

She and two assistants arrive in Zancudo on a water taxi through the mangrove channels from Golfito. For three nights they stay next to us at the thatch-roofed Los Cocos beach cabinas. We eat our meals together just down the jungle footpath at the barefoot Sol y Mar café. Our new Zancudo friends who run these places are thrilled to join in. The Costa Rican natives wouldn't know Annie Leibovitz from Annie Oakley. But to the gringo castaways, this is the biggest thing that ever happened here.

Holly and I must be the least famous people Annie has photographed. She can be blunt with her assistants, I see. But she's fun for us to work with. One day while we're walking the beach she spots an old washboard in the surf and gives it to us as a house-warming present. Holly styles it into a work of art, taking a collection of dolls' legs that we've found along the beach and dangling them from a wire strung across the corrugated tin, so they dance in the wind like chorus girls, clicking their heels.

The following winter, we first take up residence in *La Palapa Pequena*, which encloses all of 400 square feet.

I make an office for myself in a front corner of our property, behind the driftwood-piled beach. All it takes is two rubber-coated hammock hooks and two tree trunks standing 11 feet apart. The office's floor is a carpet of beige sand. Its roof is a layering of palm fronds. It will survive any cyclone and can never be broken into.

I rake away the almond leaves and fallen coconuts to configure a floor space. I drag a driftwood stump over to use for a table. Atop the stump I place an empty notebook, a new pen, a steaming cup of Costa Rican coffee, a wooden pipe full of brainstorming mixture, and a butane lighter. I fetch my hammock from the front porch and string it up. There! My Latin American bureau is up and running.

I snap a photo of the scene (minus the pipe) to show to the editors in New York who made this possible. Then I stretch out in the hammock, and I'm so tickled with myself that it takes quite some time— *boy, is this good coffee!*—to start thinking up the great novel I came here to write.

Day after day, week after week, I lie in the hammock squinting up at the shuffling fronds, and yet I do not receive any of those overarching literary visions I thought would appear to me once I left behind the distractions of the greater world. We have no TV here, no newspapers or magazines, no phone, no internet. That was the whole idea, wasn't it?, to get away? But here's what I'm discovering: I need that input. I was trained as a newspaperman. My talents as a writer—and maybe not just as a writer—lie in interpreting events, not initiating them.

At a café I find a two-week-old Miami Herald sports section and study the spring-training stats of Marlins rookies I've never heard of. I hunch over a short-wave radio, an addict, trying to pull in the Voice of America.

As an expatriate novelist, I'm a flop. But Holly finds subjects of interest in our everyday life.

In the afternoons, when the wind picks up, she takes her hammock out to her own set of hooks and settles in with a notebook and pencil. She writes picture books for children and has sold three of them to Simon & Schuster. Now she casts our beach house as the main character:

In the yellow yawn of afternoon, a tropical wind rolls off the sea. It carries the heat from the sun, the salt from the waves and the leaves from the almond trees. It twirls around the coconut fronds, turning them into a flock of fans—all feathery and fly-away. It rocks the porch and knocks at the door of Beach Shack, the snappy new hut with the shiny wood floor, solid and stable down to the core, the happiest-house-on-the-beach shack, built out of heartwork and dreams.

She writes another story about the gardener's daughter who comes over to play with her, and another one about the old woman down the beach who sells tortillas.

When I write, I try to impress editors and agents. Holly, I think, writes more to please herself.

Zancudo's beach is so level that at high tide the water laps up against the roots of the palms, and at low tide the bare sand stretches seaward for hundreds of feet, with hardly a stone to mar its end-of-the-world innocence.

The sun comes up at 5 in the morning. That's when I run every day, when the air is still cool, barefoot down the surfline through the rippling shallows. There's never anybody else around. The few houses are tucked back into the greenery, so that all I can see ahead of me is jungle and beach, sea and sky.

Holly has her own rhythms. The spiritual stuff first, then the jogging. Before breakfast, we slip into the ocean together while the surface is still breathlessly flat. She swims for the exercise. I ride waves for the fun. This life is a life lived wholly outdoors. Afternoons are for reading books (and dozing) in our hammocks on the porch. How effortless it is for us to be alone and together at the same time. How easy it is to do without friends.

Little do we know: Those photos that Annie Leibovitz took in December, 1994, captured us at the very pinnacle of our earthly good fortunes. Because it's during these first weeks of living in Zancudo, in January of '96, that Holly begins to feel that telltale trembling in her fingers.

1997
Stalking Leif Eriksson

We have crossed over the Great Divide—from before her diagnosis to after it.

In retrospect, we made the right decision to build the beach shack. That certainly might end up being our last big adventure together. Unless you count the Parkinson's.

I investigate the disease diligently, like a good newsman, to find out what lies ahead. It only depresses me. At the age of 55, I can foresee no other outcome than to be a lifelong hostage to my lover's gruesome decline.

We can't talk about it yet: our future. She doesn't want to. I envy her for being able to deny, for thinking she can escape the only truth we have left. I'm a guy who lives for the future: always dreaming up trips, trying to peek around the next corner. Now we don't have a future. No wonder there's nothing to talk about at dinnertime.

Then, at home in the mountains, we do talk.

She asks me, "What good would it do to worry?"

"We shouldn't worry," I agree. "We should just be aware. Of what's down the line."

"How would that help?"

Maybe I should just tell her: I don't want to carry the entire burden myself.

She points out, "I don't have hardly any symptoms."

I nod. "Most people wouldn't know."

"Why should I think about the future?"

"Because it's unavoidable!" Doesn't she get that?

"But it's not *here*!"

"Well..." Technically, she has a point.

For twenty years, Holly has been working at living in the here and now. Every weekday morning she puts in 45 minutes of hatha yoga, then sits for an hour of Buddhist meditation. Twenty years! Occasionally I'll mock her disciplines when I catch her doing something really unspiritual, like not loving me sufficiently. Now, I hear myself puzzle: "Maybe you're right."

She says, "We can work on things when they come up."

"Sure." I'm dazed by this switcheroo.

"Whatever comes along, we'll have to deal with it."

"Sure." What happened to all of my resolve?

To live for the moment: I've heard it said a million times before. It's so wise, it has passed into platitude. Yet why haven't I given it any consideration here? If you have a disease you can't fix, isn't the best revenge to live each day to the max before destiny lowers the boom?

Isn't this actually the same health strategy—willful obliviousness— that I have practiced all my life?

I take comfort, I take refuge, in my work.

Maybe I give marijuana too much credit. But there's nothing I love more than to kick back somewhere by myself, and get stoned, and think up a kick-ass assignment.

As a travel writer, I specialize in stories which are rooted in journalism. I like turning a dry issue into a colorful trip which brings it alive. The spectre of global warming takes me from flooded villages in England to rising seawaters in the Bahamas to glaciers going drip, drip, drip as I kayak across Alaska's Prince William Sound. The issue of global water rights takes me from the source of the Euphrates in the mountains of northern Turkey, downriver through Kurdistan by military escort, then across Hafez al-Assad's Syria to the Iraqi border.

Holly joins me on the trips which are oriented more toward tourism, like seeing Bali or houseboating the canals of Ireland or trekking the mountains of New Zealand. She stays home when I go off to play journalist.

Now what? Here I go glooming about the future again: How much longer will she be able to travel with me?

Two years? Five years?

How much longer can I leave her on her own?

The millennium is approaching, and one angle entices me. The year 2000 will be the 1000th anniversary of the Vikings' discovery of America. I like snooping around Scandinavia, and this tale of mayhem and enterprise remains strangely untold in our country—about the outlaw murderer Erik the Red and his four children, who became the first Europeans to set foot in the New World.

The drama is recounted in two Icelandic sagas written in the early 1200s: *The Saga of the Greenlanders* and *Erik the Red's Saga*. The action begins in 960 A.D.: "There was a man called Thorvald, who was the father of Erik the Red. He and Erik left their home in Jaederen, in Norway, because of some killings and went to Iceland..."

In Iceland, Erik killed again, twice, and was banished twice. To be a bane among Vikings: How bad could a man be?

He sailed away with his wife and children, including his son Leif, to a huge unknown island west of Iceland, an endless expanse of snow and ice. He named it Greenland—"because people would be attracted to go there if it had a favorable name." So he was a real-estate scammer, too.

The sagas say that in the summer of 1000 or 1001 Leif sailed west from Greenland with 35 men. In time they came to a place they called Vinland, for the grape vines they found. Here the salmon were larger than they'd ever seen. "In the fine weather," the sagas recount, "they found dew on the grass, which they collected in their hands and drank of, and thought they had never tasted anything as sweet."

Leif and his men wintered in what is now Newfoundland, or possibly in Massachusetts. In succeeding years, three of his siblings led further expeditions. But none of them stayed, or we'd all be Gunnars-sons and Gustavsdottirs.

How best to tell this story? I consult my pipe. What if we told it backward? What if it began at the ruins of a Viking outpost in New-foundland and traveled back in time to the shore in Greenland from which Leif set sail, then to Iceland where he was born, then to the town in Norway which first banished Erik, setting in motion all that came after.

It shapes up to be a three-week trip. It's one of those stories—not really sightseeing—that I'd rather do on my own. Holly won't mind. She likes being by herself. We've always granted each other breathing space.

Hell, I don't want to stay home fretting about the future. I want to live for the moment, too.

The trip begins on the stony shoreline of a bay at the northern tip of Newfoundland. This is L'Anse aux Meadows National Historic Site. Some low turf ruins upon a heath. Some ancient objects of iron and bronze inside a museum.

The land is spongy and bouldered, lichen-encrusted, with clumps of gnarled, side-blown balsams. In June the winter snow still hides beneath the rocky bluffs. Three wind-sculpted icebergs float as if at anchor in the bay.

The ruins stand back from the beach, straddling a softly flowing river that must have served the settlers well. The remains are bare-ly more than ankle-high, tracing the outlines of eight buildings—for blacksmithing, for woodworking, for ship repair, for sleeping.

It's a gorgeous day in June, the afternoon sun hanging constant in the sky, nobody else here. An excellent time, methinks, to get out my traveling pipe.

As I stand in what used to be a doorway, I realize: This is the same scene Leif took in. Out across the water the icebergs could be ships coming in, their sails driven white. One iceberg calves, breaking up in slow motion with a long-delayed clap. Then silence again. A bird crying.

Looking out to sea, it's hard to tell which shapes are islands and which are ice; hard to know what was here a thousand years ago and what will be gone tomorrow.

Getting off the small plane at the Narsarsuaq airstrip in south Greenland, I am welcomed by swarms of mosquitos.

The land is treeless and patched with snow, like in Newfoundland, with icebergs again dotting the sea. Low clouds hang over Eiriksfjord. Inuit women walk past the one hotel carrying freshly picked herbs from the hills. Inuit teen-agers lounge in the hotel's lobby, nothing to do. The long day dissolves into a static twilight until midnight and beyond.

In the morning I take a boat across the fjord with a Danish guide. Here the hillsides are green, dandelions popping up everywhere. The houses of the native sheep farmers are painted mustard and crimson and blue, lending cheer to a landscape which is usually blank-solid white.

This was where Erik the Red made his farm. We come to a bas-relief monument of him standing at the prow of a Viking ship, his arms thick, his beard and hair thrown by the wind. Then we reach his homestead, named Brattahlid, on a terrace overlooking the fjord. More ruins of turf-and-stone walls. A river rushing down from the hills.

Again I pause in a doorway and get high and gaze out upon the ocean blue. Again I'm keen to the fact that I'm standing in Leif's shoes. He was about ten when his family came here from Iceland. No wonder this rocky shore looks like the homesite he picked out at L'Anse aux Meadows.

If the Norsemen couldn't keep their culture alive in far Vinland, they made up for it in Iceland. Here, in the world's northernmost nation, live the descendants of the Vikings, going by the old names, speaking the old tongue.

Magnus Hjartarsson, who drives me in from the airport, traces his ancestors to the 10th Century, to a man so ugly he was named Skin of Hell. Icelanders know their sagas well. Magnus recites a few lines from the warrior-poet Egill Skallgrimsson, who started killing when he was 6:

My mother said a ship and fine oars
should be bought for me
that I should go off with Vikings
stand up in the prow
commanding the valuable craft
then put in to port and slay a man or two

Reykjavik is a capital of crisp lines and clean air. Statues to the ancestors are everywhere. The big hilltop monument to Leif Eriksson shows him full-lipped and clean-shaven, a battle-axe in one hand, a cross in the other.

Dr. Jonas Kristjansson, a gnome of 74, is the world's foremost authority on the sagas. I am honored to have him as my guide, riding shotgun, as I drive to the Snaefellsnes Peninsula to pick up the scent of Erik the Red. Jonas is cradling a 1935 edition of Erik's saga. His own ancestry, he says, goes back thirty-five generations to King Harald Fairhair, who united Norway in 872, then settled Iceland.

We drive north through huge glacial valleys sweeping up to ridges pocked with snow. We come to a park where Egill the lyrical warrior buried his two murdered sons. A sign conveys his words of grief:

Small prospect now of poet-god's plunder
no light-drawn load from heart's deep lair

We drive farther north, following place names from the sagas, to the Haukadalur Valley. A sign points up a gravel road: EIRICKSSTA-DIR, 8.2 km.

Oddly, Jonas has never been here. Now, brimming with excitement, he reads from the saga in his lap:

"Erik cleared land in Haukadal and built a farm at Eiriksstadir. Erik's slaves then caused a landslide to fall on the farm of Valthjof at Valthjofsstadir."

I drive up the valley. At 8 kilometers we stop at a house for directions. The old farmer, Arni Benediktsson, climbs into the back seat. He tells us his people have lived here forever. He tells me where to drive, shows me where to park. He walks us up a clumpy hillside. He turns and points across the valley to an escarpment.

That, he says, was where Erik caused the landslide to happen. He points to where Erik's slaves were then killed by Filth-Eyjolf. He points to where Erik in turn killed Filth-Eyjolf and also, for good measure, Hrafn the Dueller.

Arni leads us farther up the hill to some rectangular traces of turf walls. They look very much like the ones I saw at L'Anse aux Meadows and Brattahlid.

Old Jonas rejoices: "Now we come to the ruins!"

Can this be true? We step over the walls. Can we really be standing in Erik the Red's living room?

The site is unmarked, unknown, unprotected. Jonas paces off the single living space, twenty yards long. He wonders: Where was the kitchen? Where was the pantry?

Only later, as we're driving away, does it dawn on me.

"Wasn't that Leif Eriksson's birthplace?"

The sagamaster checks his sacred book. He calculates back through the ages. Then in triumph he proclaims: "The room where he was born!"

2004
Night Frights and Crocodiles

Seven years have passed. The Parkinson's is stealing her energy, dimming her smile. But that's not the worst of it. In 2002 she resolved to quit her medications because they were making her paranoid and delusional and causing heart-valve problems in other people. Neurologists remain addicted to drug therapy, so we started working with an alternative healer in Santa Cruz. At her advice, we dialed down the meds very slowly, over the course of ten months, to avoid a severe withdrawal reaction.

Ten months! And yet the day after she took her last pill she started having nighttime terror attacks.

Every night, around midnight.

"*Tom!*" Her voice urgent, frightened.

A minute later: "*Tom! Please!*"

Trying to rouse myself: "What?"

"Tom!"

"What?"

"Help me!"

Groggy: "Help you what?"

"Tom!

"I'm right here! What?"

"Time!"

"Huh?"

"Time!"

"Tom," I correct.

"Tom! Help me!"

"Help you what?"

"I'm dying!"

"No, you aren't!"

I couldn't get through to her, couldn't reach her. I kept trying to make some rational sense of it. Did she need to go to the bathroom? Did she need to walk around to clear her head? Was it a bad dream?

"Tom! Please!"

Turning on the lights: "HOLLY! WAKE UP!"

She was taken, possessed, neither awake nor asleep but in some inaccessible badland in between.

She'd squeeze her eyes shut like a child. "Turn off the lights!"

I'd stalk around the bed and haul her upright so she was sitting in front of the light. "HOLLY! WAKE UP!" She'd close her eyes tighter. One night I took my fingers and tried to pull her eyelids apart. What was I doing? I ordered her nonsensically: "WAKE UP AND GO TO SLEEP!"

She was someone I didn't know, this midnight Holly—hostile, belligerent. I was harsh and impatient myself. A couple of times she took a wild swing in my direction, and in the mornings both of us woke up feeling abused.

Neurologists tell us that a drug-withdrawal reaction wouldn't last this long. They say this is Parkinson's and will only get worse. But they've been wrong for us before. And sure enough the terror attacks, after two years, are easing up.

Another drug-withdrawal nightmare has stayed with her: disabling sensations of hellacious heat.

These aren't hot flashes, she swears. If I take her temperature, it's always normal. But to her the heat is real—a dry, burning, searing, roasting heat, a furnace blast, all-enveloping. At its worst, she squirms in agony. She's cowed by its power over her. When she's in its throes, I can only try to distract her with a meal or a TV show or, best of all, a puff on the pipe.

Since quitting the meds, she has been tormented by a whole galaxy of freaky hypersensitivities. Sometimes she feels "tingly all over."

Or "chafed." Or she feels "electrical zaps." Or like water is coursing through her body. Or she cannot tolerate certain fabrics or clingy clothing. Or her female parts feel "pulled" or "stretched" or "splayed" or "on fire" or "rubbed raw."

At different times she has let me know:

"I feel like a metal ball is rolling around inside."

"...like they've stuffed me with stucco."

"...like they've poured concrete into my body."

"...like my skin is being turned inside out."

"...like I'm getting pulled over by a blizzard."

"...like tiny boxes are holding me up."

"...like my waist has gone down one level."

"...like my underpants don't travel at the same speed."

This drug withdrawal is far worse than anything the disease itself has thrown at her. She is overrun with anxiety. Every day is a high-wire act. I can't dare let myself feel how awful our life is. Yet after two years of this torture she is gradually calming down, cooling down.

An exciting assignment during this harrowing period would be a welcome diversion for me. But since 9/11 the travel-writing business has taken a dive. Magazines have lost ad revenue and are handing out fewer assignments. The biggest reason I can't hit the road, of course, is that I'm anchored at home with Holly.

So far it hasn't weighed upon me too heavily. Seizing time for myself hasn't been at the top of my list. I guess it's the Detroit in me, the Midwesterner. I come from two lines of hard-working German immigrants who didn't waste time looking around for special favors.

I'm glad I don't dwell on how much I'm missing. It surprises me that I could set aside my own priorities so easily. I guess the reason I'm not dying for a break is that I see this as the most important assignment I've ever been given: to help us write a future for ourselves.

Still, an opportunity will come along once in a while that's hard to pass up. That would apply to any excuse to knock around the Australian Outback. I hear that a new railroad line is being opened from Alice Springs north to Darwin, and I notice that it roughly follows the route of the first white man to traverse the continent, in 1862. Couldn't a modern adventurer get off the train and pick up the explorer's footsteps and follow them to the sea?

Who would stay with Holly? We are past the time when she could handle an outing like this. So I'm jazzed when her sons agree to relieve me for two weeks.

These trips are so stimulating that bringing dope along is somewhat redundant. But I go by the maxim that a guy can never have too much heightened awareness.

In preparation for Australia, I go to the drugstore and survey the trial-sized bottles of shampoos. I need one with a wide mouth, one that I can't see through. I choose Helene Curtis ThermaSilk Conditioner With UltraHold.

At home I measure out the right amount of dope. I roll it up tight in self-sticking Saran wrap, slip it into the bottle and, with the eraser end of a pencil, plunge it to the bottom. The displaced conditioner overflows—all the better for masking the buried scent.

When we went to Italy in 1999, the Saran wrap leaked, making the dope damp and soapy-tasting. Still, it worked. What a romantic trip that was: Italy. We went to bed in each other's embrace every night. Those Parkinson's drugs (sigh!) did have that one beatific side-effect.

While she was still able to travel, we seized every opportunity. That same year, '99, two years after her diagnosis, we went on assignment to the Philippines to take part in a Habitat for Humanity build-out led by Jimmy and Roslyn Carter. The climate was withering, and it was tough work putting up cement-block walls and metal roofing. Jimmy was the first man on the jobsite in the mornings; no mere photo op for him. But my hero was Holly, who labored on even though her energy was flat-lining and the airline had lost her luggage. For a onetime fashionista, wouldn't a lost wardrobe be the ultimate meltdown? No, she just styled my extra pants and shirts into a raffish Our Gang look and trucked out to the job.

I'm nervous about taking dope along on this Australia trip. The scene keeps playing through my head:

I approach the customs agent in Sydney with the studied nonchalance I've perfected over years of petty smuggling. I smile at him. I offer him my suitcase and (uh-oh!) he takes me up on it. Now he's opening it. Now he's pawing through the toiletries...

Maybe I shouldn't put it in the suitcase, after all.

I examine the jeans I'll be wearing. In the rear, under my belt, is the leather Levi's patch. With a razor blade I could slit the threads on one side and create a cavity, then sew it back up again, couldn't I?

I consult the guidebooks. *Lonely Planet* says the Aussies are "extremely efficient" at finding contraband. *Let's Go* cites drug-sniffing beagles in orange jerseys. *Moon* reports German shepherds nuzzling tourists' crotches.

"What's in 'ere, mate?" the customs man asks, holding up the Helene Curtis. Doomsday. My magazine career is finished. Should I call home? My stepson Scott would pick it up. Scott the straight arrow, who likes to play the father to my wayward child. "Scott," I have to tell him, "they're sending me home on the next plane."

Packing for Australia, I flash back to the Midnight Express moment I suffered when Holly and I did Ecuador.

We were flying out of an airstrip near the Colombian border after canoeing a tributary of the Amazon. The plane started boarding, and we got in line. Then I noticed that passengers weren't walking directly to the plane. Soldiers were herding them together in groups so that dogs could smell out their carry-ons.

Oh, brother.

One of our river guides had given me two joints. They were sitting loose in my daypack. Our line kept moving forward. The soldiers weren't paying attention. Couldn't I act like a befuddled old fart and just merge in with the gaggle of passengers who'd already been inspected?

Yes, I could. I made my move, and I got away with it.

Then I heard Holly call out from her place in line:

"Tom, we're supposed to go this way!"

Busted. I rejoined the line. My life was over. I pictured what sort of jail they'd have in this shithole of an oilworker boomtown. I wouldn't last one night.

The soldiers had us circle up and place our bags at our feet, so there'd be no mistaking whose was whose.

The dog came around.

He sniffed.

He sniffed again.

He moved on.

The last time I flew to Australia I breezed right through customs. But that was four years ago, a long time. Holly was well enough to stay on her own. The twin towers were still standing. Now the Aussies are fighting with us in Iraq. Airport security is jacked up everywhere.

Maybe I can ship the Helene Curtis—send it in a padded mailer to my Sydney hotel, stamped HOLD FOR ARRIVAL.

No, those customs agents weren't born yesterday.

I remind myself of all the trips when I didn't pack dope and had a fabulous time anyway. I remind myself that I'll be traveling with guides in the Outback. Why would I want to skulk around hiding something? It would only make me feel apart from them. Why would I want to spend even one second deciding when to get high and where to get high?

After all these years of smoking, I know how it works. If I bring dope, I'll use it up. If I don't bring it, I'll forget about it.

Yet in the end here is the difference marijuana makes:

I enjoy those trips I take straight. I always bring back a good yarn. I don't notice a big difference—until I get home. Then before too long I'll fire up my pipe, and within minutes, within seconds, dazzling new dimensions to the story will reveal themselves, whole new associations, deeper connections, as my own experiences of the journey melt in with the objective certainties of journalism.

What a thrill it is when all the pieces come together like that.

This Australia trip might not be a miracle cure for Parkinson's, but as I sit on the flight from LAX to Sydney dreaming away the fourteen hours (the Aussie movie on the seatback screen, the Aussie shiraz on my tray, the Aussie fever in my brain), it's magic enough for me.

I don't have a cell phone. I won't be calling home. I am gone now. I have set my watch ahead for Down Under time. I won't even know what day it is in California.

This is my fourth Outback expedition, and the first two days are a picnic, riding trains through the deserts from Sydney west to Adelaide, then up to Darwin, looking for kangaroos and camels and brontosauruses. The emptiness is mesmerizing: a Western without actors, a land unmarked by aspiration. The Ghastly Blank, they used to call it.

In Darwin I'm met by my guide Mike Keighley, who's a buddy from past adventures, and we set out driving through the bush to pick up the trail of the explorer John McDouall Stuart. We overnight at the Bark Hut Inn, a pub whose oddities include an endangered rodent living in the tunnels of the pool table. The pub is owned by Tom Starr, my other guide, who once caught water buffaloes for a living.

In the morning the three of us take off in Mike's Land Cruiser, with a swamp buggy riding behind in a trailer. We head north on red gravel roads, then dirt tracks, through woodlands and swamps. Wallabies bound away to let us pass. A big-horned buffalo stares us down.

Soon the track becomes flooded and Tom decides, "This does not look too flash." We clamber onto the swamp buggy, and I have the best seat—perched on a plywood deck hanging out over the front wheels, with the tropic wind in my face, the water surging over my ankles, the grasses thrashing my legs. Huge egrets and herons are winging out ahead of us. A boar sees us coming and vanishes into the trees. Tom shouts in my ear, "You're first in the line of fire if we run into a croc!", and I wonder: Why am I not afraid? I could die right now, and I wouldn't care.

Finally, we're on foot. A dark patch of jungle is all that separates us from the northern sea. We fight our way through tangled branches and vines beneath the tentacles of enormous banyan trees. In every clearing, Tom makes a skid mark with his boot to help us find our way back out.

Then we come to a vast bog which has to be crawling with croc-odiles, and we can't find a way around it. We have no land left, no choice but to turn around. Mike muses, "With all our technology, we couldn't do a Stuart."

But the game is not over. As we're retreating later in the swamp buggy, a helicopter flutters down and lands. Tom knows the pilot, a rancher's son. The kid is using the chopper to herd cattle, as they do up here.

Mike sidles up to him: "D'ya suppose you could run my mate here"—he gestures my way—"over to Point Stuart?"

Mike peels off a hundred, and the cowboy reckons that he can do it. When we lift off, he banks us so steeply I'm dangling out the doorway by my seatbelt. He skims along a few feet off the ground, then pulls up just in time to clear the trees. I'm shrieking: More! More!

We fly over the banyan forest, and at last the sea is in sight. He swoops to a landing and leaps out, leaving the rotor whapping. He runs off into the jungle, and I chase after him, sweaty notebook in hand. We crash through branches and vines, ducking, stumbling, tripping, falling, swearing, laughing. God, but I love Australia! How many trips like this is a guy allowed to have in one lifetime?

He stops in his tracks, and here in the forest stands an obelisk. It's inscribed: "On this spot on 24th July, 1862, John McDouall Stuart, explorer, had the letters JMDS cut on a large tree after his successful crossing of the Australian continent from Adelaide to the sea."

Mosquitos are dive-bombing us. "Fuck!" the cowboy yelps. "No wonder Stuart didn't stay here!" And we beat it back to the chopper.

Whether or not I take marijuana with me on a business trip, there is one constant: I will write the story stoned.

Everything I've written for publication since the Ivan Arnold story in 1972 I have written under the influence. It's how I have trained my brain. I believe that it gives me an edge as a writer, helping to make up for an otherwise limited imagination.

When I try to write without dope, the phrases that come to mind just don't interest me much. They are used phrases, clunkers borrowed from someone else. I don't have anything new to contribute. It goes way back with me, since before I ever heard of marijuana—this belief that day-to-day reality, on its own merits, isn't compelling enough without some alterations.

When I write stoned, the words that flow out of my fingertips feel fresh from the oven, newborn, uncensored. They dance—or at least I see that they have the potential to dance. I can teach them to dance. They invite me to join in the suspense of arranging them across the stage in just the right order. I'm down on the screen with them, directing them, shuffling them around, bringing in new darlings for tryouts, marrying some and divorcing others: beseeching them to all sing together in harmony.

Writing is hard work. Dope is my refresh button. It opens up my tired eyes, lets me see old material with a new innocence. It makes the job more fun. The more fun it is to write, the more fun it'll be to read.

Pipe Dreams

2005
A Spark of the Divine

Janice Walton-Hadlock is a master of Chinese medicine who believes that Parkinson's is not a brain-chemistry disease but an energetic malfunction brought on originally by a childhood foot injury. The unhealed injury, she says, has reversed the flow of "chi," or electrical current, in the Stomach Channel between the foot and the brain.

Every month for four years we have driven north to Santa Cruz to spend a couple of days in the hands of Janice and her avid young assistants. It's an easy drive up the coast—four and a half hours, no big cities, no traffic. But today Holly is plagued by her out-of-whack withdrawal sensitivities—to the inner feelings of raging heat, to the sunlight falling across her lap. She insists that we turn around. Instead, I pull over and give her a puff on the pipe. This soothes her, and we drive on.

Janice's initial remedy for the reversal of chi is to repeatedly hold the injured foot in a gentle therapeutic caress known as *yin tui-na*. Once this corrects the energy flow, she says, then other "blockages" appear—old injuries and also old patterns of negative thinking and "emotional wariness" which seem to hold the Parkinson's in place.

Does this describe Holly? She was never a negative thinker. But "emotionally wary?"—that could fit. She doesn't cry. She keeps her emotions under wraps.

"In many cases," Janice writes, "the PDer has created a condition in which he feels as if he is not mentally or emotionally associated with his injured body part, or even, eventually, his own body," which inhibits dopamine release and nerve activity between the heart and the brain. "For full recovery, any attitudes that cause emotional emptiness must be overcome and new emotional habits put in place."

Janice is an ample, eye-glassed woman of 50 with a big merry laugh. She's a three-ring circus, quoting Western medical studies, Eastern mystics and philosophers of all stripes. She is open-minded and tunes in to what we say. She treats us like allies and friends. She is so involved with Holly: so partisan, so intimate, so not like a doctor.

We pull into Santa Cruz and check into our usual motel across the street from the sea. Holly goes down for a nap, and I spend an hour in Cannabisland, walking the clifftop path, watching the surfers. I like coming to Santa Cruz: the spectacular setting, the city's undying hippie flair.

Janice thinks that the dopamine-delivery system in people with Parkinson's is merely dormant, not dead. The dopamine is there, she says; the trick is to access it. She tells Holly, "Meditation is a powerful way to increase your dopamine. A focus on the Third Eye increases dopamine and lightens yourself," whereas focusing fearfully upon bodily sensations like pain or heat will decrease dopamine.

She tells Holly: "Your body will increase dopamine if you challenge it. Memorizing poetry can increase dopamine. Kipling. Robert Service. *The Rubiyyat*...read the Arnold translation." To a neurologist, wouldn't this be nonsense? "Frances Thompson"'s *The Hound of Heaven*," she recommends.

Janice tells her, "Singing can increase your dopamine. Listening to music can increase it. Play Strauss waltzes. Play *The Blue Danube. By* the Vienna Philharmonic."

Do I believe this? What do we have to lose? Western medicine hasn't done jack-shit for us except to mess up her mind, two times— first when she took the drugs, then after she tried to quit them. I buy the Strauss CD.

At home we like to play catch with a Nerf ball. It's all instinct: no thinking required. So she's very good at it, stabbing the ball out of the air and tossing it back without the usual slowness and hesitance. Now I put on *The Blue Danube*, and our games turn into waltzes—the sweeping arm movements, the swooning violins, the French horns, the arc of the ball, these newfound graces. I remember the day we walked Vienna on our driveabout through Eastern Europe.

Back and forth the ball goes. D*a-da-da-da-dum!*

Dum-dum! Dum-dum!

Da-da-da-da-dum! "Nice catch." *Dum-Dum!*

I ask, "Remember that day in Vienna?"

A faraway smile. "We loved the modern art museum."

Holly's ups and downs remain a mystery to me. I enjoy exploring that mystery with Janice. I'm buoyed to have some hope in our lives. I love it that Janice can speak to Holly's spiritual yearnings in a way that no one else can.

Holly still meditates every day. But the calmness at her center has been darkly disturbed. I think she feels betrayed by her beliefs—abandoned by God. I'm not fluent in the language, but I can tell she's lost in a wilderness between belief and disappointment. She has invested so much into prayer, and where has it left her?

It is plain to see how the disease has ravaged her physically. The cognitive and emotional depredations are no less crippling in our struggle to have some semblance of a life. But if we have any dreams left that she might some day be able to hold her own against the disease, they will probably depend on whether she can find a cure for this final calamity: her spiritual devastation.

This is where doctors fear to tread. This is where Janice jumps in. She is a long-time devotee of the Indian guru Paramahansa Yogananda and is encyclopedically versed in other religions and in the lives of Christian saints.

When we see Janice for the first time on this trip, she tells Holly a story. She went on a ten-day retreat, and every day she said prayers for Holly, seeking guidance about what she could do to help her. But she didn't get an answer. Then a friend who'd been to India gave her a gift of two stones from the cave of a saint named Babaji who was said to have communed with Christ and lived for 500 years.

"That night in my prayers," she tells Holly, "I thanked Babaji for the gift of the stones. And I felt as if he was asking me to give one of them to you."

This was the answer to her prayers: This was how she could help Holly. So saying, Janice hands her a jagged hunk of white quartz with blood-red marbling. The story has imbued it with an aura that even a barbarian like me can detect. Janice says the stone represents Baba-ji's perpetual presence, and if Holly keeps it with her she will never feel alone in the world. She can put away all of her fears, because Babaji will always be with her.

Back in Santa Barbara, I take it to a jeweler to have it set in silver so she can wear it around her neck.

First, she puts three other pendants on the chain, three artifacts of her battered faith—a cross from her childhood friend Sheila, her wedding ring, and a token from her Habitat for Humanity work in the Philippines.

Finally, she strings on Babaji's stone, and from this moment forward, wherever she goes, she is accompanied by this conjured presence of the holy man's eternal spirit.

When we arrive in Santa Cruz for our next visit, Holly is beaming. Janice tells her, "You look really bright and clear today. Do you remember a year ago you were confused a lot, losing your focus? Do you still feel that way?"

Holly concedes, "That might be improving."

"Your focus seems like it's here in the room, clearly. There was a time when you were confused. I'd ask you something and you'd go, '*Tom?*' You'd keep asking him for the answer. Now you and I are having a conversation."

Holly is a hard sell. After four years in Janice's program, she has grown increasingly pessimistic. She sees no improvements in how she is moving. I point out that she is hardly any worse, either. But her withdrawal anxieties are so intense, it's hard for her to glimpse any optimism.

Janice asks her, "What would you say is the biggest problem right now?"

"The heat."

"How about balance? The backpedaling?"

"Bad." Then she laughs. "I have to tell you about something. My granddaughter Tabatha was walking backwards, imitating me."

Janice eggs her on, and Holly gets animated, making fun of how she stumbles backward, reaching for handholds. It looks like part of a Parkinson's comedy routine.

"You're laughing!" Janice cheers. "You're really here! This is the Holly we're looking for. This is where we're going. This shows you that we can get there. If we can do it one day a month, we can do it three days a month, and then we can do it all the time. And when you're perfectly normal and healthy you still won't be radiant twenty-four-seven, because nobody is."

Holly voices more skepticism, and Janice tells her that expectations are everything. "The current is already running well through your feet. It's just a question of dopamine, which is the most expectation-influenced neurotransmitter in the body, the most receptive to the placebo effect. If you expect you'll feel better, your body makes dopamine. If you expect you won't feel better, your body won't make dopamine. It's so tied in with the emotional and spiritual component."

She mentions a patient we've met, Beth, who has nearly recovered through this program. Janice credits Beth's high expectations. "She knew one of my students. When she was told she had Parkinson's, her response was: 'I know people who treat that.' Most people are told Parkinson's and they say, 'It's incurable! Oh, shit, it's the end of my life!' Beth never doubted that she could recover."

Holly is still not impressed.

Janice talks about the importance of will power to a person's hopes for recovery, and I ask, as if Holly weren't here, "What if someone doesn't have that will power?"

"At some point," she says, "patients have a personal responsibility to decide who they want to be. There's no therapy that's going to make a person decide to rejoin the world if they are on an emotional holiday from the world."

Tough talk. "Do some people never reach that point?"

"At that point," she says, "you get into spiritual free will, and you have the choice: How many lifetimes do you want to be neutral rather than motivated by love?"

Holly speaks up: "I feel like I used to be more motivated by love than I am now."

Janice tells her: "If anyone can pull this off, you can. At some point, that spark is going to hit your head in a way that says: 'I should be worse than I am.' Or what might be even more wonderful is you saying: 'My faith in love is so strong that I know that everything I'm going through right now is part of a plan—this thing called love.' And when it clicks in, your whole emotion will switch from concern and fear to acceptance and gratitude."

Holly says, "I feel that I have to have more of a sign that I'm getting better."

"You're being tested."

"I used to have more faith. I'd read *The Course in Miracles* and I'd cry and I'd talk to God..."

"And now you're living it. Now you're one of those people you used to read about and cry about."

Holly laughs. "Yeah. I've lost it."

"You're being sorely tested. To me, the sorest test is when you can't feel love through your body, and then to thank God for the experience, because it makes you more sympathetic to others, because it's burning off karma, because it's all part of some plan you can't under-stand."

Holly chokes out a reply: "I used to feel that."

"And you can get it back!"

"I miss it so much!" she cries, with real passion.

"It can only come from you and your relationship with God. But it's there. That relationship is there still."

It's so good to see Holly crying, weeping.

Janice soothes, "Keep saying: 'God, I know you're there. Be here with me, God! I need you! I'm not going away!' You have to tell God, 'I want your love back in my heart! I don't feel your love! I can't live without it!'"

She's speaking in Holly's tongue. Holly is listening.

"Holly," she says, "you already have within yourself a spark of the divine. Connect with God! Affirm who you are! Affirm your health! You have within you the ability to be perfect. You're actually trans-forming yourself. And that's at the core of all illness, the spiritual stuff. Demand of God that he show you the path you should take. He doesn't need to heal you, to do any cheap miracles, any parlor tricks. Tell him, 'God, show me which path I should take to get back to you.' He can't resist that prayer."

I join in: "And is my role to just stay out of the way and keep buying the groceries and cooking?"

"Your role," Janice corrects, "just like her role, is to always be ask-ing God what you should do. That's been your job since you were born, and it's always going to be your job. If God says, 'Pick her up off the floor,' do so. If God says, 'See if she can do it herself,' do so."

Holly confides, "Tom isn't used to speaking to God."

"Well, he better get busy!" is all she can say.

I press on: "I play the cheerleader. But does it matter what I believe if Holly doesn't believe it herself?"

"Forget about Holly," she says. "Have you grown in this experience of being the cheerleader?"

Enthusiastically: "Oh, yeah!"

"Okay! There you are! That's your relationship with God! We're doing two miracles here at the same time! One is, your relationship with God is growing. The other is, Holly's is growing. Some of us are lucky enough to do it side-by-side. Good! Excellent! You're at a time in your lives when most people are slowing down. You're being told, 'Come on! You've got the potential! You can do this!' Fabulous! That's what your job is: continue to grow in your relationship with God."

If I'm Holly's cheerleader, Janice is mine.

2005
Mr. Dependable

Our children, my two and her two, are in their late thirties now. We're lucky that they're thriving. They don't need to lean on us for support. They bring wit and affection and conviviality into our ever-narrower lives.

For Thanksgiving, my daughter Jenny and her husband Rich fly to Santa Barbara from Austin, and son Andy drives up from San Diego. They are bright, fun-seeking missiles, Jenny a Ph.D English teacher, Rich an advertising writer, Andy a natural-foods buyer who has gone back to school.

On Saturday afternoon, Jenny asks Holly out to get their nails done. I'm happy to see my two favorite women making like girlfriends, because it doesn't happen much.

Andy and Rich and I have never been left to our own devices. What are we going to do? With these two guys, I know where to begin. I bring out my bong.

In time we drive to an Italian restaurant that has a bocce court out back. It's in sad shape. But that's okay. We are all more playful than competitive. Later on we go to a pool hall, where Rich morphs into a pinball wizard while Andy and I shoot some eight-ball.

By the time we get home, it's dark. I'm surprised the women aren't back. Reflexively I worry: Is Holly okay? Then I remember—Jenny's 40th is coming up. I know where they are, shopping at Anthropology. It gladdens me, and also saddens me, for both of them. It reminds me of how many simple pleasures are missing from Holly's life. It reminds me that Jenny always wanted Holly to be more of a mother—to go out for lunch together, to share secrets, to get girly—but that Holly wasn't interested.

At 7:30, they breeze in with bags full of clothing. Jenny cautions, "Dad, don't look at the receipts yet."

Do I care how much they spent?

At Christmastime, Holly's side of the family comes to Santa Barbara. There are four grandchildren—two for Scott and Melissa, two for Robb and Numi. Holly is happy to sit down and let the holidays happen around her. The old Holly was a control freak who had to set up perfect Christmases for her sons. This Holly doesn't have the energy to run the show, and she doesn't try. She has not only given up that earlier self, but seemingly forgotten all about it.

Scott lives in New York and works as an investment manager for people of wealth. Robb lives in Santa Fe and is the family's environmental activist. I get along well with both of them, thanks in part to our penchant for self-deprecating humor. My relationship with Scott has been mellowing ever since he went to live with his father, where he wanted to be from the start. Robb and I enjoy a sense of kinship built around being younger brothers.

Last year the boys and I hit a rough spot when we met in Charleston for Holly's 60th. For the birthday girl, the excitement of the occasion brought along its wicked stepsister, anxiety, and that satanic ally, The Heat. Her body stiffened; her shoulders ached; her arms jerked. She spent most of the time in bed, the boys fussing over her.

It was a disaster. Both sons got angry. They accused us of "dropping the ball." They said we were making bad decisions, weren't taking care of ourselves. As Scott put it diplomatically: "YOU GUYS ARE BLOWING THIS BIG-TIME!"

They grilled us about why Mom shouldn't go back on the drugs like the doctors kept telling her to do, and why we weren't signing up for brain surgery. The way Holly was acting, I couldn't claim any progress. They didn't want to even hear Janice's name. I argued that these symptoms were caused more by the drug withdrawal than by the Parkinson's. I argued that the surgery, like the drugs, could make her mental deficiencies worse. But they didn't want to hear any of that. All they knew was that their mother was going down the drain unless they rode in to save her.

Anger intimidates me. It was one of the countless emotions I didn't run into growing up. When I'm under attack, I clam up and get teary-eyed. So the boys talked us into setting up conference calls over the coming weeks with the country's leading deep-brain neurosurgeons.

We phoned doctors in New York, Miami and Cleveland. Their opinions varied—about whether the operation could further imperil a weakened mind, about how permanent the bodily improvements were, about whether the procedure was advisable for all Parkinson's sufferers or just late-stage patients looking for a Hail Mary.

The split decision gave me some breathing room. I followed up in good faith by taking Holly into Los Angeles for a neurological exam that the surgeons recommended. A diagnosis of dementia would rule her out for the operation, and I was half hoping for that result—to end the debate.

The examination was a two-hour interrogation by a psychiatrist who must have trained at Guantanamo Bay. Poor Holly. She knew what he was testing her for. Dementia had always been her biggest fear. She barked out the answers to the shrink's questions like a Marine at Parris Island, her forearms pumping away like jackhammers.

She ended up passing the test. Meanwhile, however, her sons have backed off of their campaign for the surgery, their zeal to intervene. They can see she's more composed since her birthday. They have their own dramas at home to attend to. They know that, as Holly's lawful health-care agent, I get to make the final decisions.

I'm so relieved to be rid of that political pressure. I can't ever force Holly to choose between her boys and me.

The brothers might react impulsively and challenge me when they see their one-and-only going downhill. But I can tell that their gut feeling toward me one of gratitude, for how I've taken care of her while they've been busy raising their own families. Whatever happened between us in the past, I have ended up being, if not their mother's guardian angel, at least her unblinking servant.

They understand that I'm their last line of defense.

Three days after Christmas, on my 64th birthday, the two laddies treat me to a round of golf at the area's most spectacular course, Sandpiper.

It's laid out on the bluffs overlooking the Pacific. The day is warm and sunny. Robb is a good golfer, while Scott and I spend our afternoon stumbling through the rough looking for balls gone astray. The brothers are sharing one cart. I am happy to have my own. Every four or five holes I drive off into the trees where they can't see me and take a puff on my traveling pipe.

God, what a beautiful fucking day this is!

When I line up a shot now, it's so easy to picture the flight of the ball...rocketing sky-high...plunking down in the middle of the green. So what if the shots don't turn out that way? I can still have fun driving the cart.

We reach the 11th tee, a par three from an elevated tee to a green nestled beatifically down along the beach. I get ready to tee off. Then the boys call me over to the bench. It seems they've devised some kind of ceremony.

Decorously, they sit me on the bench between them. Robb reaches into his golf bag and pulls out three Jack Daniels miniatures. Scott, the family historian, who studied at Oxford and Cambridge, thereupon delivers an eloquent toast proclaiming that the positive attitude I display in the face of adversity is the same spirit that made the United States a great nation.

I protest, but not strenuously. I'm flattered.

We down the Jacks. They pull out three Coor's to celebrate our Colorado heritage. Then we play on, the holes running along the ocean cliffs while the sun sets behind us. Looking for a lost ball, I have another toke.

We have come so far, the three of us. When I moved in with their mom, I was a nonperson and they were collateral damage. But seasons turn. Holly can't be the mother she once was. The adoration between them is stronger than ever, but now it's the boys' turn to nurture her. As it happens, their dad is also in neurological decline. They're in the same boat with him.

The upshot is that, after a third of a century on the fringes of a family that I didn't join until the end of the play's first act, I've been given this opening to take on a more responsible role, and I welcome it.

I am pleased with myself—Tommy the bad boy, Tommy the wife-leaver, Tommy the irresponsible, Tommy the outrider, Tommy the joke-monger, Tommy the free spirit, Tommy the hippie, Tommy the stoner—I'd delighted that I have ended up becoming a Mr. Dependable to my own two storm-tossed children and to Holly's sons, as well.

2006
The Dope Doctor

One morning I drive Holly to her annual appointment with Santa Barbara's marijuana doctor, David Bearman.

Under California law any physician can prescribe medical cannabis, but at this point in time very few of them are willing to. So Dr. Dave takes up the slack. He's a sixtyish walrus of a man with a raspy voice. The first time we came here I saw a statue of the comic-book freak Mr. Natural on his bookcase and figured we wouldn't have any trouble getting approved.

Bearman seems well-intentioned but scattered. Today his receptionist isn't in, so we wait out front while he fields phone calls. I page through *O'Shaughnessy's*, a periodical devoted to cannabis legalization. I fiddle with a toy on the table that's filled with undulating gels, like a lava lamp. Dr. Dave is old school.

This is our third certification visit with him. It's old news by now that a puff on the pipe can smooth out some of Holly's anxieties and drug-withdrawal quirks. When she gets stoned I usually notice a softening of her demeanor, from high-strung to more or less collected. Her physical therapist, who's no druggie herself, won't work with Holly unless she's relaxed (i.e., medicated).

Dr. Dave calls us in into his office. He asks Holly how her tremors are compared with a year ago, but the dialogue doesn't flow. Bearman is hard of hearing, while Holly is soft of speaking.

I translate: "Marijuana doesn't help her symptoms directly. But when she's less anxious she usually moves more fluidly. Most days she takes just a puff or two."

"Why not more often?" he asks, not knowing which one of us to address.

I give her a chance to answer. Then I volunteer: "She's afraid for her lungs."

Bearman suggests using a vaporizer instead of a pipe. He gives me two studies showing that even long-term pot smoking causes no increase in cancer and might even have properties which protect against lung cancer.

He tells Holly that marijuana's therapeutic effects last for three or four hours. To treat the anxiety most effectively, he says, she should follow that schedule. But she isn't buying it. She's always been leery of crutches, like her mother was. She has a history of going to doctors and then not doing what they tell her to do.

The meeting over, Dr. Dave launches into a review of state and federal efforts to reform marijuana laws. He can see that Holly wants to get going. So he alternately expounds, then apologizes. But we know the drill: You have to sit through his political talk to get the certificate.

He finishes, and I reach for my wallet. He likes to be paid in cash. He tells me he has raised his fee to $200. "But since this has been such a short meeting," he revises, "let's make it a hundred." I know he feels sorry for me, for having to deal with Holly.

I give him $150. "You do good work," I tell him.

I help Holly to her feet, and we walk out hand-in-hand. In the waiting room I see the next patient. He's another senior citizen who lives in the area, someone whose name would come up if you Googled rock-and-roll drug busts. There's no mistaking those white shocks of hair straggling out from under the baseball cap: David Crosby.

Bearman's letter of approval advises: "Because of the uncertainty of the application of federal law, I cannot suggest to you where you might obtain cannabis, and I do not by this recommendation intend to encourage you to engage in any illegal activity."

But I know where to go. Of the half-dozen Santa Barbara dispensaries, I patronize the Compassion Center, whose two storefronts are conveniently down the street from the Trader Joe's stores where I buy our groceries.

I walk into the office on upper De La Vina Street, which is nestled between Jack's Kitchens and Jake's Cottage Cuisine Café. The waiting room is more inviting than Dr. Dave's, with potted plants, vases of flowers, an Indian tapestry, a sitting Buddha. Jazz is playing. On a shelf: a stack of the pro-cannabis *Oaksterdam News*.

A muscular black man in a tank-top is waiting. What can be wrong with him? Is he a caregiver, too? The door to the inner office buzzes. A bald man emerges with a paper bag in hand, and the bodybuilder goes inside. A young guy walks in from the street with a skateboard. He phones a friend to say, "I just got my cast cut off."

Most of the customers I've seen are men, not notably well turned out. The most common complaint is said to be chronic pain. The *Oaksterdam News* quotes one doctor: "No other drug works like cannabis to reduce or eliminate pain without significant adverse effects. It evidently works on parts of the brain involving short-term memory and pain centers, enabling the patient to stop dwelling on pain."

Cool! The same thing that makes us dopers forget what we're talking about also lets us forget that we hurt.

I leaf through a ring-binder titled *Strain Guide*. The Cinderella strain is labeled "uplifting and giggly." New York City Diesel is "good for making or enjoying art." What works for washing dishes and taking out the trash?

The black man emerges with his bag. I enter, and Mara takes my new paperwork from Dr. Dave. It authorizes the Compassion Center to grow a certain number of plants and to enroll me in the "growers' club." At harvest time, I'll get two ounces, worth about $700, as my share.

I scan the blackboard for today's specials. The full ounces are Bubba Kush at $400 and Trainwreck at $380. The menu also lists dessertified medications. Marijuana Brownies. Rice Krispie Treats. Chocolate

Pecan Truffles.

I get an ounce of Trainwreck because it promises more of a head trip than the body high of the Bubba Kush. Mara puts it in a paper bag printed with old-fashioned ads for snake-oil remedies. Careless packaging, if you ask me.

When I return home, Holly is still napping away. I get out the inlaid wooden pipe I bought at a street fair in Woodstock, New York. I tear open the metallic pouch of Trainwreck and put a pinch into the bowl. Holly is the one with the license, but I'm the one with the appetite.

I flick the lighter. Inhale.

Preventive medicine.

The helper's healer.

Exhale.

The Old Samaritan's energy source.

Instantly I'm bristling with the illusion of robust well-being.

2006
Reveries of Foie Gras

The San Ysidro Ranch outside of Santa Barbara, where producers and princes hide out, where JFK and Jackie slept on their honeymoon, has been fixed up since the last time we came here. I used to park my own car. Now a sign warns of folderol ahead: valet parking. I surrender our dirty Subaru to the kid. For sure, he'll notice the sweet aroma inside. I walk around to help madame climb out.

It's the evening of my 65th birthday, a year after that game of golf along the ocean. We are here to dine at the Stonehouse Restaurant, courtesy of my stepsons and their wives. The hostess leads us through a dark lounge with a potbelly stove like one at a lodge in the Tetons. Then we're shown into the dining room, to a good corner table.

This is always awkward, getting seated. First comes the decision about who sits where—me dedicated to pleasing her, she protesting but finally succumbing as the hostess stands waiting for a resolution. Tonight I direct Holly toward the pillowed nook that looks back into the room instead of the chair facing the wall. She insists that I choose tonight, and I accept the justice of this.

The act of sitting is further elongated by Holly's disabilities. She is not able to lower her weight slowly while scuttling crabways into position, then land her butt squarely on the cushion, then scooch the chair up to the table—a complicated series of feats. Instead, I pull the chair back and guide her into place (*nudge-nudge*), until she plops onto the seat. I reach down to muscle the chair forward over the carpet with a snatch-and-grab, scrape-and-haul effort that I won't always be able to muster. Lastly, I seat myself. Only then does the hostess step forward with the menus, completing the introductory floor show.

I'm wearing an Orvis travel-guy jacket over a blue Ex-Officio travel-guy shirt that I bought for myself today. I like this look—me ready to take off on some big adventure. How sad is that? But why did the hostess ask if she could hang up my coat? Does she think it's an overcoat? Have I missed the mark for this fine establishment?

Holly is in her calm, comfortable, composed phase so far, her hands resting inconspicuously on the tablecloth. Ergo, I'm relaxed. Since her hair appointment last week, she is radiantly, photogenically blond. If there are any people in the room who didn't see us laboring to get seated, they are wondering now: "What's a doll like her doing with that old buzzard?!" They're guessing: "She's a gold-digger and he owns some travel-sportswear chain."

The waitress brings a dish of Mediterranean olives to awaken our palates, then a dish of radishes. The menu is short. I spot a tortilla soup. Holly is fumbling through her little Holly purse for her reading glasses.

The next appetizer, Grilled Foie Gras with Toasted Brioche, Stone-Fruit Chutney and Balsamic Vinegar, triggers one of my habitual travel reveries.

"Remember that restaurant in Denmark?" I prompt her. "Where we had foie gras steaks? That country inn?"

"Did we bike there?"

"Along back roads, yeah."

"Through the grounds of a castle," she remembers.

The memory expires. The appetizer, I see, costs $19.

We are both frugal, even if we hail from different constellations. Her sons told us to forget the price and order whatever we want tonight. Still, nineteen bucks for an appetizer? Instead, we decide to share an arugula salad that's $13. "It's healthier," I justify.

I'm relieved when the ordering is over. Holly hasn't seized up with indecision, as she can. She hasn't proposed some off-the-menu brainstorm. No, it's me who's second-guessing. I'm chiding myself for passing up the foie gras.

Isn't this supposed to be my night of nights? Hasn't Scott, who manages Holly's family money, urged us to spend more on ourselves? Isn't that why I splurged on a Gillette Fusion five-blade razor today? "Prosperity consciousness," we used to call it in the hippie days. Isn't that a worthy goal for a late-bloomer like me?

The difference between those appetizers was six bucks. That's $3 a couple for the boys and their wives. Or $1.50 a person. Or 75 cents if you include their kids.

I return to wallowing in the reverie: Denmark, 1993. We were so charmed by that country inn, the Falsled Kro. It was on a tidal inlet. We walked around the shore in the evening, the sun in June way high in the sky. Then dinner at the best restaurant, it was said, in all of Denmark.

I spot our waitress and catch her eye. "Would it be too much," I ask, "to get the foie gras *plus* the salad?"

She reasons, "It's your birthday, isn't it?"

The fabled dish arrives at the table, and I try a corner of it. "Like brie," I croon. I give Holly a taste. The portion is small, and as I'm nearing the end of it I try to make each bite exactly half the size of what's left on the plate, so it will last into infinity: my foie gras, my receding memory of Denmark, my veteran life.

The waitress brings complimentary sips of Lillypilly, an Australian sauterne. I love Australian wines, for one reason: They stir up memories of traveling there. With every sip, a voice whispers in my ear: *Remember Australia?*

Holly raises her glass shakily. "Happy birthday, sweetheart."

I lift mine and catch the sparkle in her eyes. I want to rejoice: *Hey, everybody: Look at that smile!* At one point she was losing her facial expressions—taking on the frozen mask of Parkinson's. I noticed it when she wore sunglasses, how her cheeks looked fallen, immobile. Now I don't see that as much. Sometimes I wonder: Have I merely gotten used to the mask? Tonight, I believe.

We work our way through the entrees and the dessert. Then the waitress brings one last thing: flutes of Nivan. She says it's a vanilla-infused cognac from Madagascar, and that triggers still another travel memory—trekking through the jungle with that famous primatologist.

I ask Holly, "Remember Madagascar?"

"The lemurs," she recalls.

"The beggars knocking on the car windows," I recall.

"What was her name?"

The primatologist, she means. "Patricia Wright."

We decide to drink the Nivan in the other room, by the fire. I wrench her chair sideways to clear a pathway, then help her to her feet. With my free hand, I toss down the last drops of her $13 glass of pinot grigio.

It has been a great evening. We have gone out into the world of glamor and position and conducted ourselves almost like normal people. All of my life I have yearned to be seen as different. Right now, I'm liking normal.

For a long time I have understood that even on a day like today that's all about me, it's still mainly about her. Despite my history of ducking obligations, I seem to have been groomed from Day One to be the giver of care in this minuet, while Holly was destined to be the receiver.

We walk out into the cold night air. Blondie feels it to the bone, and I wrap an arm around her. Our car wheels up, and the valet kid hops out. I help her into her seat.

We pull away, and I can already feel the heartburn coming on. Ahh, yes, the foie gras.

I don't remember this happening in Denmark.

2008
Mr. Nobody

Every autumn we drive across the country and back. I have come up with this notion, based on discoveries in the field of brain plasticity, that the novelties of traveling might stimulate Holly's neurons enough to slow the advance of her disease. At least it can't hurt her. I love the open road, and she's contented to ride along as my hostage.

Eleven years after the diagnosis, her ability to express her thoughts is eroding. Her movements are slower and more hesitant—but not a whole lot. I'm with Janice: Shouldn't she be getting worse faster than this? To me, she's on a plateau. Is that just wishful thinking?

The best news is that she has pretty much outlasted those agonies of excrutiating heat. Her whole complex of hypersensitivities has gradually lifted, like a fog. So that <u>was</u> drug withdrawal. Six fucking years of it.

When we're on the road, she starts each morning in our motel room with a reduced regimen of meditation and yoga. I figure that it's safe to leave her alone for an hour. So I go out to take an exercise walk.

I used to always prowl the local historic district. But that came to seem like a knee-jerk approach which was too exclusive. Now I usually leave my prejudices and my car keys behind and walk in our own neighborhood.

Sure, any hike that begins and ends at a Hampton Inn or a Wingate Suites is going to cover terrain which is brutally unnatural and desecrated. But isn't there some value in the practice of seeing the world as it is?

Besides, I take my morning walks stoned. So one setting is just as enthralling as the next.

A good time to light up is while I'm descending the motel's bleak concrete stairwell, which is always deserted. I emerge into the parking lot and exhale into the morning light. Then my trek begins as this expanse of bare asphalt gives way to the next one and the next, past Quik-Marts and Quiznos and Long John Silver's, past Family Dollars and Dollar Generals and payday-loan shops.

While Holly is making herself a better person, I'm scuffing past old soda cups and cigarette butts, getting my fresh air with a chaser of exhaust. I hike through the shadows of the KFC bucket and the Arby's hat, then back into sunshine again. I troop through the Honda dealer's lot, the Accords posing with their engines warming up and their doors flung open like a chorus line. I pass a Speedy Joe's and a Papa John's, an Old Navy, a Rib Crib Barbecue and a Supercuts, their parking lots separated by paltry no-man's-lands of spoiled grass.

The Chrysler dealer is yahooing its monster year-end closeout. Old Glory ripples overhead. The loudspeaker calls: *"Kurt Brand on two!"* Balloons bob and weave in the stiff prairie wind. *"Kurt Brand on two!"* Salesmen eye me through the windows, not a customer in sight.

I pass a cineplex whose marquee says CLOSED. A Jiffy Lube with its bays standing empty. An abandoned department store whose sign has been removed but whose name, HOMELAND, stands out in clean lettering against the dirty façade.

Weeds poke up through cracks in the pavement. Dead leaves scurry past. I puzzle over a bird's wing lying next to a crushed pink barrette. I picture these shopping strips as future ghost towns in some post-consumer America.

Then the human spirit makes an appearance. A message board in front of a dentist's office spells out, WELCOME HOME SPC. JESSE WATKINS, and gives his phone number in case we want to call and wish him well.

This is my beat now, and it's one more unexpected gift, one more victory over ghastly probability. Even if I'm just working the seams between one shopping mall and the next, I am where I most want to be: anywhere but home.

As a writer I am always pleading to be shipped off to Tashkent or Timbuktu. Now I'm glad that, as fate reins me in, I don't have to go to the ends of the earth to have experiences that will open my eyes.

As the Chinese master said: "The Great Way is easy for those who have no preferences."

When I get stoned, the preferences fall away.

On a Saturday we pull into Bardstown, Kentucky. Holly is hoping to spot some lovely old inn which feels like a B&B but doesn't force you to eat breakfast with strangers. I settle on the Best Western because it has a morning buffet that we can eat in the privacy of our room.

Over time, she has withdrawn from human interaction—partly, perhaps, out of embarrassment for her condition, but more out of a simple loss of interest, a grand turning inward. Even when we're on the road, she manages to remain a hermit, and I am her enabler. I drive her from one motel to the next, from door to door. I bring our meals in. I can't imagine another couple living like this.

The Best Western is one of those old-fashioned motels where you can back your car right up to your door. I help her get out, and she shuffles into the bathroom. I carry our luggage in. I put her bag on the dresser where she can reach it without stooping. I unzip her toiletries kit and hang it over the sink. I prepare the bed for her afternoon nap by taking off the spread. She hasn't touched a hotel bedspread in ages, since she saw a semen-on-the-quilt expose on *Dateline NBC*. I prop up three pillows for her. She flops onto her back, and I help her get positioned.

She asks, "Could you tell the front desk to bring us more pillows?"

I decide, "We've got enough pillows."

"They don't mind if you ask."

It's an old discussion. She is an orchestrator. I am an adapter. I like to make do with the pillows we have rather than take the trouble of arranging for more. If I call the front desk, how long will it take for the guy to bring them by? I'm itching to go take a walk.

She tries again: "Couldn't you ask for more pillows?"

I kiss her on the forehead. "I'll take care of it."

Note to myself: Pick them up later at the office.

She already has her eyes closed. I sneak out the door like a burglar, patting my pocket for the key. Now is when my time begins. She'll be fine for an hour or more before she needs to get up to pee. Meanwhile, as soon as the door clicks shut, I am free. And it's the best kind of freedom: a freedom I am grateful for, because it's so rationed.

When I'm out walking the sidewalks of some town I've never set foot in before, I can be certain that no one who sees me can possibly know me, and no one who knows me can possibly reach me. What a godsend it is for the caregiver, to have this fleeting opportunity each and every day to be Mr. Nobody: unneeded, unwanted, untouchable, invisible.

I duck behind a bush to do that illegal thing which augurs to make the walk that much more gripping. Then I drift down into Bardstown. It's only a few blocks, and my mind can either tag along or take off on its own.

The leaves are falling. We're heading back out west. This is our fifth cross-country trip in three years, and it's been the easiest one yet for her. How would the neurologists account for that?

We are on the road so much, I can lose track of where I am—what town we're in, or what state, or even what part of the country. I'll be gassing up the car or sitting at an Applebee's ordering a glass of wine and two dinners-to-go, and I'll wonder: Is this Maryland? Ohio? Missouri?

Then in Bardstown my Mr. Nobody shtick goes too far.

I'm on a side street approaching the main drag. I glance up and fix upon a red-brick facade basking in the slanting sunlight. Then my mind goes blank—my whole memory—not just of where I am, but who I am. My whole story: gone.

For an instant it's exhilarating, to escape. Then I'm panicked not to know: *Who am I?*

It's like I've fallen down some deep, dark hole, and I'm clawing for a handhold, for a way back up to the light. Then I see an image—of a room with a woman lying on a bed.

Yes! I know where that room is! It's behind me and two blocks over. Yes, I know that lady.

The panic eases. Now I remember who I am. I'm the man who has to get back to that room to look after that lady.

Once I understand that, the rest of my story falls into place: the writer, the father, the fool. Ah, yes.

Does it bother me, that Holly and her disease have hijacked my identity so completely? That my selfhood has nearly disappeared into the black hole of codependency?

No, all I'm wondering is: Do I need to get back to the room yet?

I look at my watch.

Hey, lucky me. My walk has just begun!

2009
Hostage Crisis

Zihuatanejo, Mexico.

Holly and I pull up to the *aeropuerto* in our rental car. We're re-turning from a family Christmas vacation, and I'm furrowed with re-sponsibility about the flight home. I get out of the car and set out to perform my tasks, in the right order.

First: strap on my daypack.

Second: haul our overstuffed suitcase out of the trunk.

Third: position myself outside her door with the bag propped against my rear leg so that after she steps out we can start walking im-mediately rather than having her wobble around precariously while I grope for our belongings.

Fourth: open her door and unbuckle her seat belt.

Fifth: assist her in exiting the vehicle.

But, dammit!, as her left foot reaches out for the curb, her sandal (the one I figured would be easy to slip off at security) falls into the gutter. She is poised half in the car and half out of it, and we execute a bumbling little tango, me with one hand in the small of her back and the other hand swooping down to try to get the thong of the sandal, *dammit!*, between her toes.

The tensions of air travel are savage enough even for the ful-ly-equipped, so when I was planning this trip I went into Mother Hen mode. I asked in advance about security lines for the disabled. We spent the night before leaving L.A. in an airport hotel that had a shut-tle bus straight to the terminal. Still, shit happens. In Mexico now, as in L.A. a week ago, I waltz through *Seguridad* while Holly has to put up with all the pat-downs and body scans. A granny with Parkin-son's?...the perfect Al Qaeda cover.

The anxiety of flying seems to mess with her balance. On the flight to Mexico she got her legs crossed on a trip to the bathroom and fell into my arms. After we landed, she faltered again descending the stairs to the tarmac.

Now, climbing back up the stairs, she takes a misstep and teeters backward. I steady her and murmur profoundly, "One foot after another, honey." Then she makes up for it by leaping up, miraculously, two steps at once.

Before we take off, an attendant reads a list of new rules from the Transportation Security Agency. While we've been in Mexico, the Nigerian underwear bomber has tried to blow up a plane entering the U.S. So we're told that for the last hour of our flight the bathrooms will be locked.

Oh, brother.

Soon after we get airborne, Holly signals that she has to use the toilet. It's the best of news—going now rather than later. I help her to the bathroom and lean into the cubby to turn her around.

I warn her, "Don't lock the door. I'll be waiting right outside." I picture her getting locked in, banging on the door, the whole crew mobilizing to help the oldsters out of their jam. "*Don't lock the door!*" I repeat.

No such disasters ensue. The mission is completed, and we return to our seats. Immediately, she falls asleep.

Ahhhhhhhhhhhhhhhh. I picture how great it's going to feel to be back in our car in L.A., back in control of my destiny, driving up to Santa Barbara. I picture fishing my pipe out of the glove box and taking a hit of medicinal hash to make the drive home that much more illustrious.

"LADIES AND GENTLEMEN!" the attendant announces. "WE HAVE TWENTY MINUTES LEFT UNTIL THE BATHROOMS ARE CLOSED!"

My hostage is still fast asleep. I study her face. It's a judgment call. I think she'll be okay.

"LADIES AND GENTLEMEN! YOU HAVE TEN MINUTES BE-FORE THE BATHROOMS ARE LOCKED FOR THE REMAINDER OF THE FLIGHT!"

Maybe I should wake her up.

"LADIES AND GENTLEMEN, FIVE MINUTES TO LOCKDOWN!"

Now there's a line-up for the toilet. I don't want to make a scene. Hey, she'll be fine. I nod off myself.

Eventually, we begin to descend. I look out to catch that stirring sight of Los Angeles sprawling from horizon to horizon. Then I see my Holly stirring awake, too.

I squeeze her hand: "Almost there!"

She says something I can't hear. But I can definitely read her lips: "I...have...to...go...to...the...bathroom."

I gaze out the window, imagining the many humiliating ways this could play out—in the aisle of the plane, in the jetway, in the customs line. Our descent takes forever as we swing out over the Pacific half-way to China.

I picture the two of us making a rush for the plane's lavatory—being tackled and handcuffed and stuffed into overhead bins.

Tomorrow's headline:

Continence-Challenged Seniors
Held in Airline Toilet-Bomb Scare

The plane touches down. Holly is pretty composed. It's me who's a wreck. I'm the quintessential caregiver: I've taken on all of her anxiety for her.

We taxi—WHERE THE HELL ARE WE GOING?—to the farthest edge of the most remote runway. Here we wait for a month and a half. I warn the steward: "You're going to have people peeing and crapping all over your planes!" He agrees: "The TSA always overreacts."

At the terminal, we make it to the immigration melee without shaming ourselves yet. We come to a maze of crowd-control strapping, and I call out to an officer: "My wife is disabled and can't wait in line!" He unhooks a strap, and I charge through the opening like a blocking fullback, right in front of a mother with her children.

She starts to protest, and I wheel on her: "MY WIFE IS DISABLED. IS THAT A PROBLEM FOR YOU?"

She backs away in horror.

Crazed Caregiver
Held in LAX Brawl

The immigration clerk stamps us through and points out the restrooms. I tug Holly over there and let go of her hand, and the momentum carries her through the doorway.

Whew! I fall back into stakeout mode, loitering near the doorway like a stalker, watching women come and go.

I wait for her. I wait for her. I wait with mounting consternation that I might have to take some action. What am I supposed to do? I'm not going to just barge in there.

Presently a customs officer comes up to me and asks, "Are you waiting for your wife?"

Is there a look in the eye?

"Yes, I am."

"Are you Tom?"

Uh-oh!

The bathroom has two doorways, it seems, half a mile apart. My honey has been waiting outside the far exit.

I hustle down there. Then I see her in her straw bonnet, standing tilted to one side, clutching her little Holly purse. She breaks into a pretty smile when she sees me, and a whole new wave of affection washes over me.

We take a taxi to the Doubletree Hotel, where our car is parked. I'm thinking about the hash pipe that's waiting for me in the glove box, and about how I deserve it because I didn't take any dope to Mexico.

At the parking garage, I do everything in order. Pay the driver. Done. Put on my daypack. Done. Get our bag out of the trunk. Done. Station myself outside Holly's door. Done. Open the door and assist milady in exiting the taxi and finding her balance. Done. Done. Done. Kick the cab's door shut. Done.

In the garage, I help her into the car. Done.

I get into my seat and reach over to pull her belt across her lap. "Want to buckle it?" I invite.

She gnashes the fittings together unsuccessfully. I wait. I wait. I put the hash pipe in my pocket. I wait.

At last...*click.*

"Good job!" I cheer, Coach Tommy.

I start driving down the corkscrew ramp, the tires squealing giddily. Then I realize that she's trying to say something. Her voice is so soft, it can be hard to tell.

"Huh?" I inquire, too loudly, leaning her way.

"Those chocolate...?" she whispers.

"What?"

Silence. Then again, "Those chocolate..."

I hope she's not talking about those chocolate-chip cookies the Doubletree has. I'm dying to hit the road.

"What is it? Just say it!"

She yells: "THOSE CHOCOLATE-CHIP COOKIES!"

"OH, COME ON!" I cry, like I've been stabbed.

"Just two cookies? It's such a long drive!"

Whatever her cognitive gaps, this woman can recall the taste of every chocolate-chip cookie she has ever eaten.

I whine, losing traction, "Can't we just drive home?"

"Please?" she begs.

Sighing, I park in the hotel's unloading zone and go inside. Oh, great!—some South American soccer team is crowded up to the counter checking in.

I catch a clerk's eye and call out, "Cookies?", waving two fingers like I'm bidding at an auction.

"We ran out! A new batch is coming in ten minutes!"

I wave my hand. "Don't bother."

The princess will have to do without.

I walk outside and stop to take in the damp evening air. It is scented with sweet expectation like the first time I ever came to California, and I'm glad to be back. I stick a hand into my pants pocket, and it comes into contact with that talisman, the dope pipe. Inevitably, this leads to a realignment of my thinking.

What's the big hurry, anyway? Why can't I be a good guy and wait for that new batch of cookies?

I stroll around the corner of the hotel.

This way, she'll get 'em fresh out of the oven.

I find a darkened doorway and duck into it.

Tomorrow's headline:

Brazilian Footballers Tackle
Old Doper in Hotel Bomb Scare

Each giant Doubletree chocolate-chip cookie comes in its own paper slipcase. I escort her two back to the car, one in each hand. They warm my upraised fingers. I like pleasing people, pleasing Holly. So I'm disappointed in myself when I grunt like a weary slave, "Okay, here they are!", as if I didn't delight in my little walkabout.

I pull away, turn onto Sepulveda, and blow past the entrance to the 105 freeway that I meant to take. But, hey, I don't mind. The surface streets will do just fine. I'm still on Mexico time. On maryjane time.

As I drive on, I have a gathering awareness that Holly is sitting there fingering her two cookie bags—not trying to open them, just fondling them. What's up with that?

Finally we get sucked into the freeway system, joining the chase up the 10 to the 405. The traffic is ballistic. I have to kick it up to 75 to jump lanes. We're in a rocketship, hurtling through the million-and-one lights of an L.A. Saturday night.

I glance her way, to see that she's still feeling up those cookie bags, as if she's nursing a critical thought about them. I should just stay out of it. Instead, I ask her: "Don't you want to eat those cookies, babe?"

She has a question of her own, her foggy voice lilted with girlish longing: "Are there two in each bag?"

An old weakness of mine, for gratitude, kicks in. "Can't you just be glad for what I did bring you?"

I take the 405 north to the 101.

She whispers, "I'm sorry."

I lean over and squeeze her knee. "I'm sorry, too."

We don't have to say what for.

Finally, on the Ventura Freeway, the traffic thins out. For the first time all day, I can relax.

My hostage, I see, has fallen asleep.

I relax two more notches.

Ahhhhhhhhhhhhhhhhhhhhh.

She had a good Christmas. Her grandchildren enjoyed her. Nama, they call her. Earlier in her disease, she was worried that the kids would think she was "weird." But they accept Nama for who she is. Whimsical. Vulnerable like they are. Spellbound.

She is sleeping soundly, her head bobbing forward, her hands resting at peace by her sides. In her lap are those two empty cookie bags, her souvenirs of the trip home, plus some good-sized crumbs that she must have overlooked.

The Unlived Life

2011
Seized

Where am I?

I am lying in a bed, on my back, in a white room, bright lights drilling down from above. I'm straining to breathe through a tube stuck up my nose.

Where am I?

Is this a hospital?

A doctor leans over me. He looks like my son Andy.

Maybe he isn't a doctor.

"Andy?" I croak, fuzzily.

"Hi, Pops." Reassuringly.

Where am I? What happened?

It happened yesterday morning, I am told.

Yesterday. All I remember is how it began: helping Holly get up... guiding her to the bathroom like any other day...helping her sit on the toilet...wiping her. Later her physical therapist came over, freeing me for an hour. I went out to my office, opened the door...

Then one last memory: waking up on the office floor, my face covered with blood.

I have to be told what happened next—how I drove to a doctor's office to get stitched up...how I drove to an MRI clinic to check for a concussion...and how, in the lobby of the clinic, I fell to the floor and thrashed around in the thrall of a grand-mal epileptic seizure.

Whoa!

Let me step back for a minute.

I have to tell you.

It has been a hard year.

We spent last summer, the summer of 2010, in Colorado, as usual. At first, Holly's old women friends raved about how well she was doing, how good she looked, how full of vigor. Then in the middle of July she crashed. It started one night when four of us went out for dinner and she felt ignored. Quickly the insult escalated: She thought her best friends were laughing about her behind her back. At the same time, she was falling apart physically—losing energy, needing much more help to get around, plunging into a severe bout of diarrhea, getting dehydrated and feeble.

I was overwhelmed. I needed more support, and I made an executive decision. After the summer we were moving to Santa Fe, where her son Robb lived with his family.

We drove down there on Labor Day. We rented a cute little casita in the old-town arts district and stayed for the winter and into the spring. It was good to have family around. But Holly was still failing: physically, mentally.

We weren't used to the cold winters. There were no sidewalks for our exercise strolls. The roads were slushy. We missed California. We missed working with Holly's physical therapist. The casita was charming, but it wasn't home. The furnishings...the pictures on the walls...the reminders of another couple's great adventures.

In May we celebrated Mother's Day with the family, then packed up to drive back to Santa Barbara. I no longer trusted Holly to go into public bathrooms on her own, so I looked online and found some heavy-duty diapers that women glider pilots wore to contain their fluids on long flights. Thus equipped, we got into the car in Santa Fe and I drove the 400 miles to Flagstaff nonstop at 85 miles an hour. The most stressful trip of my long traveling life.

Day 2: nonstop to Barstow.

Day 3: bat-out-of-hell home.

Three weeks later: the seizure.

Soon after I wake up in the hospital to see my son's shining face, the doctors unplug me and set me free.

Later I have an appointment with a neurologist. Given what Holly has been through, I couldn't be blamed for not wanting to get near a neurologist. But I'm scared.

The most terrifying moment of my otherwise untraumatic childhood came when I was 12. I stood watching through the front window of our family cottage on Saginaw Bay as my father went suddenly berserk in the yard—yanking around crazily in a lawn chair, toppling it over, arms and legs flailing. My grandmother cried: "Marv's having a heart attack!" Aunt Jo yelled, "Somebody get a clothespin!"

The next day he came back from the hospital and assured everybody he was fine. The doctors said it was just a heat stroke. But when he looked at me I saw something new in his eyes, some vulnerability, some fear.

Months later back in Detroit, at the dinner table one night, he blacked out—dropped his fork with a clatter, his face all ablank. "The Bay!" he kept insisting. "THE BAY!" Then he snapped out of it—picked up his fork and kept on eating, as if nothing had happened.

Later, Mom tried explaining it to Jerry and me. "A petit-mal seizure," she called it. I hated these strange new words. Plus, she told us, Dad had suffered two more of those thrashing-around attacks in the middle of the night.

For months afterward, I lay awake in our attic bedroom at night listening for noises downstairs, dreading that at any time, at any moment, he might start going crazy again. What if he swallowed his tongue? I was petrified that I'd be called upon to take some decisive action to save my father's life.

My neurologist is a young guy with a casual manner. I'm afraid about my future, but he tells me he likes my chances. Many people, he says, have only one episode. He prescribes a medication, Keppra, for safety's sake. I know I'll take it devoutly, out of the same fear my father felt.

He tells me he's suspending my driver's license for six months. He advises me to take showers and not baths.

I ask, "You mean baths can cause seizures?"

"No. But if you had one you could drown."

Couldn't I die from falling in the shower? Suddenly risk is around every corner, atop every staircase.

I ask him if I should go to the ER if I have another seizure. He says that if I'm not injured I can just pick myself up, dust myself off and keep on trucking.

"Great!" I say, not wanting to picture it.

Finally, I ask him about marijuana. I fess up that I do it several times a day and it's an integral part of my being. He doesn't act alarmed. Maybe he's a doper, too.

He suggests, "Why not try cutting down to three or four days a week." Hardly the condemnation I'd expected.

"Great!"

That evening I sit down with Holly to try to have a conversation. We're at the dining-room table, in our usual seats. After Santa Fe, we're happy to be in our own house. She has perked up some, being back here.

I take her hands in my hands. I don't always know if she's comprehending what I say. Sometimes she can't manage to speak.

I say: "Honey, I've been taking care of you for all of these years." Pause. "And I'm going to continue to take care of you." Longer pause, to let it sink in. "But now I have a problem of my own that I have to deal with."

It's a historic occasion. It's what my friends and children—even Holly's sons—have been urging me to do. I have to get out from under some of this burden. I have to start taking care of myself. I have to get a life.

She is nodding her head, as if she understands.

2011
Don't Think Twice

The Santa Barbara Bowl is an intimate outdoors arena on a wooded hillside at the edge of downtown. We have lived in the neighborhood for twelve years—so close that we can hear the music from our deck. Yet we've never gone to a concert or even considered it. Holly rarely ventures anywhere, and I—out of equal parts loyalty and laziness—haven't taken the initiative to do much on my own. Now look at me. I have a seat up front, and Bob Dylan is here.

The setting sun is illuminating the eucalyptus trees towering above the stage. Through the live-oaks I can see out over the city's red-tile roofs to the traffic along the 101 and beyond it to the blue Pacific, with its sprinkling of oil rigs and the Channel Islands on the horizon—all the beauties and blasphemies which make California a dynamic destination still, even for those of us who live here.

It has been twenty-nine days, and counting, since my double-whammy seizure. I considered giving away tonight's ticket and staying home, where I feel safer, even if Holly couldn't manage to dial 911. I pictured going grand-mal at the concert—no one to help me, no one to comfort me. Me, the big world traveler: afraid to leave my own house.

The band assembles onstage. Then the hairy little god-creature appears, juking out from behind the curtains in a flat-brimmed straw hat and a zooty black suit with sideburns and that wimpy mustache and his hard-times Dylan mug. He steps up to the keyboard and calls out all stagey and gravelly:

It ain't no use to sit and wonder why, babe,
It don't matter anyhow...

It takes me back to 1972. To my heartache Linda. The Linda who let me go but then wanted to hold on. The Linda who sent love letters to Colorado over the years, pining to see me again. The Linda who ended up in Key West, tending bar. The Linda who died one night at 36 when a car ran her down while she was riding her bicycle home.

Listening to Bobby's lament, fantasizing what would have happened if I had dared go to Key West, I pick up an old sweet smell in the air from over my shoulder. It's a scent, like patchouli oil, that takes me back to Linda, and I look around. Is that doobie headed my way?

Yesterday I had an appointment with a pulmonologist to talk about a CT scan that was taken at the hospital. The pictures revealed a troubling "nodule" on one lung. The doctor asked me to get another scan in three months.

"In the meantime," I ventured, "you'd probably tell me not to smoke any dope at all, right?"

"That's what I'd advise."

I pressed: "Even if the clinical trials are mixed?"

"It's better to be cautious," he said.

He had to say that; I could sue him for not saying it.

I tried, "What if I use a vaporizer?"

Now, at the concert, I'm craning my neck, looking for that joint. On my wrist I'm wearing an ID bracelet which reads SEIZURE DISORDER and lists some phone numbers to call, just in case. On my head I'm wearing a padded cap to protect my battered control panel from another concussion.

It's getting dark. A full moon is coming up from the sea through the arms of the eucalyptus trees.

It's getting dark. A full moon is coming up from the sea through the arms of the eucalyptus trees, and Dylan aches to recall when he woke up, and the room was bare and he didn't see her anywhere and felt an emptiness inside.

I have never fully let go of my enchantment with her: Linda. Holly is the love of my life; Linda was my passion.

I'm so glad that my old friend Ivan Goldman from the *Washington Post* talked me into coming to this concert. Even if the worst happened, he pointed out, what better place was there to die than listening to Dylan?

Now he sings about me, he asks about me, the blue-eyed son: Where have you been, and what have you seen, and what will you do when that rains starts to fall?

I don't want to play cautious. I don't want to die cautious. Here comes a joint, at last.

It's high time I get a cannabis prescription of my own. I have a legitimate disease now. Just in case one episode of epilepsy won't earn me the certification, I make up a Plan B: my back hurts from hauling up a disabled wife.

I see a new dope doctor, and she's happy to tell me that epilepsy is a disorder that cannabis is especially good for. "Look it up on Google Scholar," she says.

I tell her that my neurologist suggested I cut back to three or four days week.

She's puzzled. "I wonder why he'd say that?"

I assure her, "I gradually went back to everyday."

When I get home, I go to Google Scholar.

The fact is: There aren't many serious studies of marijuana's possible health benefits, because of its shady reputation and legal status and because dosages are hard to standardize. The evidence that I dig up is dated, going back five or ten years. But all of it is encouraging.

At an epilepsy care center in Alberta, 21% of the patients told researchers they'd used cannabis in the last year. Of those, 54% reported fewer seizures, and 68% said their seizures weren't as severe.

Experimental Neurology magazine reviewed the research and found: "These observations suggest clear potential for effective therapeutic modulation of endogenous cannabinoid signaling systems in the treatment of human epilepsy."

The website Europe PubMed Central published a review of the literature by a New York University neurologist, who wrote: "Although more data are needed, animal studies and clinical experience suggest that marijuana or its active constituents may have a place in the treatment of partial epilepsy."

The journal *Epilepsia* ran this interesting comparison of the effects of various drugs:

"The use of cocaine is associated with the occurrence of seizures. Amphetamines and related drugs rarely induce epileptic seizures at therapeutic doses. Caffeine at high doses may induce epileptic seizures. Psychedelic compounds rarely induce epileptic seizures, but the most common clinical complication of Ecstasy is seizures. Marijuana, at variance with other psychostimulants, owing to its serotonin-mediated anticonvulsant action, could have a medical use for the treatment of epilepsy."

A review in a pharmaceutical journal offered this assessment: "Marijuana is used in the treatment of various movement disorders including dystonia, Parkinson's disease, Huntington's disease and Tourette's syndrome. Marijuana is also used to prevent seizures in patients with epilepsy and is believed to have neuroprotective properties."

Later in the summer, I go back to the pulmonologist to get my lungs re-scanned. He tells me there is no evidence left of the nodule that he found before. I don't have to return for any more tests.

After forty years of doing my level best to abuse my lungs day in and day out, after forty years of taking weeds and stuffing them into pipes and setting them on fire and sucking the living bejesus out of the other end, I'm clean.

2012
Wouldn't It Be Nice

A year after the Dylan concert, I'm back at the Santa Barbara Bowl. Standing onstage are two surfboards, old longboards, like Easter Island totems. Above them is an art-deco "50," because this is a fiftieth-anniversary tour.

The Beach Boys are here.

I'm beaming from a dose of medical hash. A plastic glass of red wine is nested between my feet. The video screen behind the band shows black-and-white footage of boys surfing in the '60s, then a blood-orange California sun setting behind a row of leaning palm trees.

The band's opening chords are unmistakable. We know this celebration so well: about the East Coast girls and the Southern girls with the way they talk and the Northern girls with the way they kiss.

My California girl, my East Coast girl, keeps slipping farther away from us. She has been so diminished for so long, it's getting harder to remember the creative dynamo who shared this winding path with me. The artist. The poet. The author. The teacher. The decorator. The chef. The fashion stylist. The athlete. The outdoorswoman. The spiritual seeker. The yogini.

Now most of her systems—her lungs, her digestion, her circulation—are compromised and at risk, according to the nurse we have brought on board. Twice she has picked up dangerous bugs from sick grandchildren. After Christmas, she was laid low by an exhausting round of diarrhea. After Easter, she got a bronchial infection that could have turned into pneumonia.

They sing another one that resonates: How nice it would be if we could wake up in the morning when the day was new and every kiss was never-ending.

She can still walk around the block, once, with me holding onto her hand. It's the other part that troubles me. Sometimes she thinks her helpers are stealing from her. Sometimes she sees people who aren't there.

I take another hit of hash. Why shouldn't I? I want to feel my feelings to the marrow. It stirs up a whole new wave of emotions—to recognize that this caregiving job, this opportunity of a lifetime, will not be mine forever.

Over the last year, I have stuck to my pledge to get more help around the house and take more time off. While Holly was struggling with diarrhea, I was in Queensland reporting about global warming. When she was on the brink of pneumonia, I was in a workshop at Esalen.

The Beach Boys are singing about her again: about the colorful clothes she used to wear, about the way the sunlight fell upon her hair.

The life we had together was one good vibration, one excitation, after another. For twenty-five years we had the best run that any couple could have.

For me, the last fifteen years have been even more inspiring. I've gone from being a selfish Good-Time Charlie to a selfless Good-Time Charlie and halfway back again. I feel an inner glow from helping someone who needs me. I've discovered that I can be happy even in bad times.

I must have beneath me some foundation, some emotional bedrock, which keeps my mood buoyant regardless of the circumstances. Marijuana deserves some of the credit for this, sure. But not all of it. I should thank my workaday parents, for giving me a stable, uneventful, worry-free, drama-free upbringing.

I always presumed that I would make my mark in the world as a writer. Now I see that my real accomplishments have come as a caregiver, and I'm better off for it.

I am also plumped up with gratitude for having forged loving relationships with my children after fumbling the ball following the divorce. The passage of forty years has deepened the appreciation that Jenny and Andy and I have for our similarities and bonds and the roads we've taken. It has also served to ease my guilt. For all appearances, taking care of Holly has helped to redeem me. Whatever its wider toll, this Parkinson's curse has given me the chance to become more human.

2012
The Goddess

Santa Barbara's medical-marijuana storefronts, which once out-numbered Starbucks outlets, are all closed.

The Obama administration, waving the tattered flag of prohibition, has been going to war against dispensaries all over California since last fall. Some 500 businesses—all of them legal under state and local law—have been shut down through various means of intimidation.

Now, in May, the strong-arming comes to Santa Barbara. Federal agents raid two dispensaries and a farm. Other shops close to avoid being raided. Government lawyers sue landlords to seize their rental properties under civil forfeiture laws unless they evict the undesirable tenants.

The U.S. Attorney's Office in Los Angeles is proud to announce: "All known marijuana stores in Santa Barbara County are now the subject of federal enforcement actions."

Dr. Dave Bearman, long an activist in the movement, protests: "The people who are suffering most right now are exactly the types of patients that the voters of California were thinking about when they passed Proposition 215 [The Compassionate Use Act] in 1996. The very sick, the elderly and those with little to no experience with recreational use of cannabis have been left to fend for themselves. It is a truly unfortunate and difficult situation."

Where do I go these days to get my medicine?

I sit back and let it come to me, because—thanks to the feds—it's all home delivery now.

At my age, I take just a toke or two at a time. But I reawaken my genie eight or ten times a day. I run through an ounce in a month and a half, and when I'm running lean I go to the website of my dealer, The Goddess Delivers. I scroll through page after page of available strains.

Cookie Monster.

Dragon's Breath.

Yoda Kush

Blue Dream.

Black Ice.

Red Congo.

Green Candy.

Purple Gorilla.

Jack the Ripper.

Girl Scout Cookies.

Rhino Trainwreck.

L.A. Confidential.

Sour Diesel.

Key Lime Haze.

Lemon Jack.

Blueberry Trinity.

Pineapple OG.

Pussycat.

Afgooey.

What have you.

I order with my Mastercard. Delivery is overnight, and it's free. When I step out to get the newspaper in the morning, the unmarked box is cozied right up to the door.

2013
Time of Transition

Hollyhock is a retreat center in British Columbia devoted to personal realization and progressive social change. The setting alone is enough to awaken the spirit, looking out across the saltwaters of Desolation Sound to range after range of snow-crusted peaks.

To get here, I fly to Vancouver, then farther north to Campbell River, where I overnight. In the morning I take a ferry to Quadra Island, catch a ride across Quadra, then hop another ferry to Cortes Island.

Cortes gives off a retro hippie vibe that wins me over right away. The long hair and bare feet. The families skinny-dipping together. The hitchhikers. The homegrown.

Like Esalen Institute in Big Sur, Hollyhock attracts a certain amount of old malcontents from the '60s and '70s. We have to trek to the farthest, most leftward edges of the continent, it seems, to find these last vestiges of our countercultural idealism and optimism.

I have come here to attend a five-day workshop called Time of Transition, because it perfectly describes my own state of flux.

After an eternity of sharing my life with women, I'll soon be forced to take a path of my own. I've been helping Holly with her myriad physical and mental difficulties for seventeen years—a third of my adulthood. But she doesn't have much longer to go. One year? Two years, tops?

For her, and for me, it's a time of transition. I'm already starting to pivot toward solo adventures. That's why I signed up for the workshop, to give myself a shove.

We sit in a circle inside a timbered dome, a skylight drawing down the sun. Our leader is a man in his sixties, Thomas O'Kane, who goes by his Sufi title Atum. (*Ah-TOOM.*) I see the Irish lineage in his puckish delivery and twinkly eye. He has spent most of his life sitting at the feet of the world's masters of psychology and religion, and he's here to pass along their knowledge. He's a humble enough messenger, talking to us only about what he has learned and not about what he has done. He dresses casually, betrays no vanity. When he reads to us, he reads children's books. He is not a guru. He's a storyteller of the spirit realm.

On the first morning, he spreads out a deck of cards on the floor, like Tarot cards, with the picture-side up and the text-side down. Dharma cards, he calls them. He asks us to each come forward and pick one. I wait until everyone else has chosen, then scoop up the last card left: the coveted unchoice.

I can't relate to the illustration—a Hindu riot of swirling red streamers and corpulent bodies. What matters, apparently, is the message on the other side, the one message which destiny has intended for my eyes. I turn the card over. It says:

> *You are a yellow leaf.*
> *Death awaits you at the door.*
> *And you have no provisions*
> *For the journey.*

All right. Then I came here to pick up provisions.

This ordeal with Holly has had a profound effect on me, and it's something I didn't see coming. As she has grown weaker and weaker, I have grown stronger and more vibrant. I don't know how to explain it. I'm satisfied with the choices I've made for her. I haven't always been patient enough or gentle enough. But I have no regrets.

I think that any guy would mature—he'd develop a more confident sense of himself—if he had to come to terms with a jam in which he had all of the responsibilities, and his partner had all of the needs. I didn't choose to be a more giving person. I just kept answering the bell. I'm not a warrior. I didn't seize the moment. The moment seized me.

And it changed me. When I get out of Holly's orbit and mix it up with these open-hearted people at Hollyhock, I notice that I have some newfound luster, some magnetism.

What's going on? As a kid I was shy. I stuttered. I was content to be a follower. Now I see people being drawn toward me. I see that I have something to offer.

When I'm away from home, I crave what I no longer have with Holly—connection and intimacy. I turn incorrigibly playful. I'm ready to get heartfelt with whoever is game. And, true to my history, I usually give in to my instinct to crank up the exultation. Before a workshop session begins, I'll shamble off into the woods to do that thing I do to be the highest, most engaging me I can be.

The timing can be tricky. If I call upon the pipe right before a session begins, it might trip off a fugue of daydreaming at the beginning, distracting me from what's happening in the room. The same after-burst of images and ideas which makes dope a good launching pad for writing can deafen me to other voices. So my strategy is to fade back into the trees twenty or thirty minutes before a session begins, to let that initial buzz give way to the mellower, more receptive Phase Two of the experience.

Still, it can be hard to contain the euphoria.

Atum asks us: "Take. Three. Deep. Sighs."

With each sigh, I should be letting go of all of my teeming thoughts, all of my mind games. Instead, I keep congratulating myself: This was so smart of me to come here, to let myself grow into who I'm becoming.

Atum asks us to write down an answer to the question: "What is your attitude toward your life right now?" And I feel such joy to be exactly where I am—in this circle of generosity, under this sage tutelage—to be allowing myself the pleasures of this community of earnest seekers who are all undergoing their own tender transitions. Atum asks it again: "What is your attitude toward your life right now?"

"Unbridled fucking optimism," I have to write.

He asks: "What is your attitude toward yourself in your present state?"

Three. Deep. Sighs.

"Love," I have to admit.

If death is waiting at the door, it can take a number and sit down. My new life is going to come first.

Atum asks us: "What state would you like to be in when you die?"

It can't get any better than this, can it? This state of ecstasy I'm in now? With these new mates?

He asks: "What do you want to become?"

I have to confess: Only what I am now.

Is it wrong that I'm so happy with my station? Or are these the provisions I'm looking for?

Atum tempts us to consider our "unlived lives."

He says, "Ask yourself: Is there a piece of my unlived life that longs to be lived, for the sake of my soul?"

Who among us would answer "no"?

Lucky for me, my unlived life isn't in the past. It isn't some fork in the road (like running off with Linda) that I wish I'd taken. My unlived life is just beginning.

Atum lets us know: "The prison door is always open."

He suggests: "Unhook it."

He seems to be speaking directly to me, about that incarceration I am ready to be released from. But I sense that the others feel it, too—that he's addressing their own needs to escape from their own private confinements and limitations and prejudices and addictions.

Atum gives us an invitation: "Tell me a possibility."

I write: "That I am beginning a whole new life."

"Tell me a possibility."

"That I will listen to my own needs."

"Tell me a possibility."

"That I will continue to feel all the joy I feel now."

"Tell me a possibility."

We have fifteen minutes to imagine what possibilities might be lying in wait. And here is the trick. When I go over my list, I see that these aren't just possibilities, they are probabilities. And not even probabilities.

Hell, they're already happening!

On Sunday the workshop ends. We hug each other good-bye. It's hard to give up the camaraderie we've built up during our time together. While I wait for the ferry that will carry me away from Cortes, I slip off into the forest dark and fire up, in order to illuminate the way ahead.

Within minutes, the words of an e-mail, a group love letter, come raining down out of the sky.

That night I send it off.

TO: david76@gmail.com; margie@solidsystems.ca; misty@cox.net; ljmattson@comcast.net; tom@huntercox.com; jp@lummerman.ca; jack@trinity.ca; tommy@lesser.net; mallorie.jenkins@jetblue.com; nancy45@rocketscience.ca; alan@lifesupport.org; nanda@shoutout.de; trueblue@superweb.com; blake32@gmail.com; rrogers@treadwell.com; stringly7@gmail.com; ptbellweather@carmel.gov; mackie5@gmail.com

Dear New Friends:

Here I sit in Room 309 at the Coast Discovery Inn in Campbell River. I am alone.

No Alan and Diane. No David from Scotland. No Jack from Kalamazoo. No Rick from Hamilton. No Misty. No Maggs. No Nanda. No Peter and Sheila. No Julia from Munich. No Joyce. No Judith.

No other Toms but me.

Worse: No master of ceremonies. No Atum.

My hotel room looks across a parking lot toward an injury-law office, a lottery shop, a Java Shack and a Tangles Hair Salon, with only distant glimpses of the natural spectacles we came to know on Cortes.

No eagles swooping low over the beach here. No deer stepping lightly through the grass. No hikes through the woods to Hague Lake. No swimming naked in the sea.

We are scattering across the planet now. Tomorrow I fly to Vancouver, then San Francisco, then Santa Barbara.

No more poems by Rumi. No more pearls from Jung. No personal myths. No archetypes. No Reb Zalman. No Pir Vilayat. No baskets of crayons to help us give shape to our dreams. No sacred stories. No listening to our hearts speaking. No Dalai Lama. No rocking out to Aretha.

No three sighs.

No four seeds to plant for the future.

No five stages of completion.

No doors standing open begging us to leave our stale selves behind.

When I get home, I won't be telling my wife much about my week with you. She wouldn't be able to respond in a meaningful way, and it would leave me feeling deflated. So I'll keep what we learned to myself, where it is encrypted.

We are returning to earth. No more hugging strangers. No more spilling family secrets. No more fairy tales. No more picture books. No more teacher's impish looks.

Surely the intimacy that we experienced at Hollyhock is its own form of spirituality, whether we believe in a god or not. We are so much better off than we were a week ago, so much more able to begin living our unlived lives.

2013
Highway Robbery

I'm driving around the desert Southwest visiting old friends when, at the junction of two empty California highways out near the Salton Sea, I come to a U.S. Border Patrol checkpoint.

Usually I get waved right through once they see I'm just a dumbbell senior citizen. This time the agent stops me to ask, "Do you have any narcotics in this vehicle?"

"No, sir."

He motions me on toward a second man in uniform, this one being tugged forward by a nosy German shepherd. He inquires, "Do you have any narcotics in this vehicle?"

"No, sir," I repeat, truthfully.

"Do you have any marijuana in this vehicle?"

"No, sir," I lie.

He points a finger. "Park over there in Stall One."

Oh, brother.

Sitting on my passenger seat is a well-traveled wooden dope pipe. Next to it is a zip-lock bag with two cannabis-laced gluten-free cookies given to me by a crony in Sun City, Arizona. In my trunk is a small baggie containing a strain of smokeable exhilarant known as Durban Poison.

I park the car in Stall One and bounce out innocently.

"Stop right there!" an officer commands.

I freeze.

He asks, "Do you have any narcotics in this vehicle?"

"No, I don't," I swear.

"Do you have any marijuana in this vehicle?"

"No, I don't," I swear. Then I remember that I have a trump card with me, and I do a one-eighty. "Yes, I do," I declare, reaching for my wallet. "And I have a California medical-marijuana license for it."

I picture him thanking me for my forthrightness and apologizing for the inconvenience and wishing me god-speed in my golden-age wanderings. Instead, he sends me away to a roadside holding pen. There I pace in circles, worrying whether I'll ever get home to relieve the caregiver who's looking after Holly.

"Sit on the bench!" my captors order. They take my driver's license and my medical get-out-of-jail card. They ask me to tell them where my stash is, so they won't have to start shredding the upholstery.

"In the trunk," I confess. "In my suitcase. In the toiletries bag. In the front zippered pocket."

Three new detainees, Spanish-speakers, join me in the pen. I move over on the bench.

A young agent sidles up to ask me, as if out of mere curiosity, "Do you use it in the car?"

I feign disbelief. Do I drive around this awesome Western landscape stoned? At the age of 71? "Of course not!" I scoff.

Then a Jessica Chastain from *Zero Dark Thirty* takes me off to a bare chain-link enclosure. I flash back to the waterboarding scene. Are they going to strap me down and extract my THC?

Jessica confronts me: "You have been arrested before for marijuana possession." It comes out not as a question, but as a recitation of historical fact.

How do they know this?

Is it even true?

My mind reels back over the decades. Then I remember, from my earliest hippie days, when I was still writing for the *Washington Post*. "You're right," I tell her. "In 1972. In Reston, Virginia. For holding one roach."

She has no interest in my early-midlife hijinks, but informs me that my state medical card gives me no right to transport my alleged medicine through a federal checkpoint, even one that's forty miles from the nearest border. She tells me she's prepared to fine me $500 on the spot.

"But I will cut you a deal," she says. "I will let you go if you abandon your marijuana."

I ask her, just to clarify: "If I paid the fine, you'd still take the dope, right?"

We exchange tight smiles.

"That's right," she says.

I nod sagely. "I'll take the deal."

Jessica walks me to my car, explaining how this is going to go down. I will retrieve the offending baggie, and she will escort me to yonder blue dumpster, where I will personally (to make it all the more painful, I guess) dispose of my mood-altering materials.

I look through my trunk and can find no sign of the Durban Poison. Jessica is annoyed to hear this. She calls out to the other officers, "Who's got the evidence?"

One of them points.

Ah, yes. There on the roof of the car lie the baggie and the pipe, embraced in damning configuration.

I reach up to retrieve them.

Jessica offers, touchingly, "You can keep your pipe." I like where our relationship is heading.

We mosey toward the dumpster, and she turns to gab with the other agents. She's paying no attention to me. Is she giving the old duffer an opening? Is she inviting me to pocket a couple of buds for the long drive home?

No, I'm just happy to get out of here a free man.

True, I'm not totally free if they have a file on me going back forty years. True, Jessica will add this new criminal act to my record. Maybe some day when I fly in from overseas they'll take me aside at LAX and kick me around a little. Maybe they'll put me on the Most Wanted list: Grandpa Stoner.

I drive away from the checkpoint and get up to highway speed. I chance to look over at the passenger seat.

Oh, happy day!

Sitting there in plain sight, unabandoned, are those two inspirational cookies I smuggled in from Sun City.

2014
Let It Go

I am sitting in a desert canyon near Palm Springs, on a flat rock overlooking a pool of water. Palm Canyon is one of the few places in all of California where the palms are native. Holly and I used to come here when we lived in our trailer. We brought lunch, books, the *L.A. Times*. I packed in some dope, of course. We were so well matched. On hot days we swam, or just sat in the water up to our necks, bobbing along side by side, sharing the solitude.

Today's hike hasn't been nearly so relaxing. I'm all knotted up with stress. Here I am on a ten-day vacation from caregiving, yet the issues of caregiving have tagged right along. Holly's son Scott is upset that I haven't taken his advice and hired a full-time live-in caregiver for his mom. Two weeks ago he scolded me on a family holiday, and I'm still feeling insulted.

I guess he thinks my three part-time helpers and I aren't doing a good enough job. Does he know that taking care of Holly is the only way I have left of expressing my love for her? Who does he think he is, trying to tell us how to end our romance?

Yes, I've thought of hiring someone to live in our guest room and take over the routines. Thanks to Holly's inheritance, we can afford it. But I'm reluctant to give up our beloved privacy. I have thirty hours of relief a week. Isn't that enough? Maybe some day I'll step back from the front lines. But I don't like being pressured.

Hiking the canyon, I've been plotting what to say in my defense. I've composed half a dozen e-mails in my head. Now here I sit on the rock, and there's not another person in sight. This is how I've planned it. I need to be alone to look for some peace of mind.

I reach into my pocket and bring out my pipe, which I have saved for this time of reflection. After forty years, I still believe I do my clearest thinking stoned.

One puff.

Another puff.

Wow, look at those canyon walls, so finely sculpted, all caramel brown with swirls of butter pecan. Look at the palms—how the dead fronds hang down around the trunks like hula dancers' skirts. Look at the boughs of the tamarisk trees dancing in the wind.

The pale blue of the desert sky.

The reeds standing tall at the river's edge.

The mesmerizing pull of the current.

The insects joy-riding along on the surface.

Why was I blind to these miracles before? Why couldn't I see what was all around me?

Suddenly I'm not dwelling on family politics. Not rehearsing imaginary arguments. Not living in the past or the future. I am nowhere but here.

A voice comes up within me, and I speak the words out loud:

"Let it go! Let it go! Let it go!"

The instruction seems to echo back off the canyon walls, and my shoulders let go of the tension. There are no issues left, no wounds, no resentments. I know that Holly's sons are hurting. A year ago they lost their father to dementia. Now their mom is disappearing.

I utter the prayer again, less defiantly, more assuredly, feeling the words sinking in:

"Let it go. Let it go. Let it go."

When I head back to the trailhead, I feel a bounce in my step. Now my vacation can begin.

Back home, I let a couple of months pass. I want to show everybody I'm going to move at my own pace. Then I start looking for a full-time caregiver. Scott is right: It's time to call in the National Guard.

Holly is so frail and unsteady, it's too risky for her to use the steps to our bedroom. I turn her old downstairs office into a room for her. I put photos on the dresser of loved ones she might be seeing again— her parents and her brother Robin.

I put in French doors which open up to the kitchen, so she'll feel more a part of the action. But her world keeps shrinking. Twenty steps to the dining table. Fifteen to the couch where we watch the evening news. Ten to the bathroom. She needs someone beside her, to keep her from freezing in place or falling. How long will it be before she's in a wheelchair?

Her new bed is a hospital bed which can lift her head up by remote control. I hate it—the industrial steel, the grinding gears, the side rails slamming like prison doors. This is her death bed. Does she understand that?

I hire a live-in caregiver, Ruth, a former RN who has to let everybody know what a loving person she is. During the first week I notice that her memory is failing. She can't remember which supplements to put in Holly's shake. Worse, she can't remember how much Milk of Magnesia to give her. She can't remember how to get to the bank, just a few blocks away. Great! Now I have two women to take care of.

I put another ad on Craigslist and hire Bonnie, who's younger and presumably sounder of mind. But I'm a lousy judge of character. I like people too quickly. I'm too trusting. On Bonnie's second day, I ask her for a grocery list. She puts down beer, wine and Bailey's Irish Cream.

But it's all for the best. I scrap the idea of a live-in helper and go for a tag-team approach, instead: a nurse, a physical therapist and three caregivers who take turns staying overnight. A hospice commune. The women become endeared to Holly, and she to them. She will spend her final times at home, in their caring hands.

Having a rotating cast of characters works for me, too. Every day I have someone new to talk to, someone to share the poignance with, talk strategy with.

I'm less of a hands-on caregiver now than a manager of givers. I have nearly wall-to-wall professional coverage. But nobody stays long enough to get burned out, or to get on our nerves. More preciously, I have saved certain times when Holly and I can be together alone—including all day Sunday, which was always our day to get cuddly.

2014
Days of Weed and Roses

Except for some stirring encounters with Ram Dass in the '70s, I have never had a teacher, a mentor. I have not thought to look for one. Now I'm going all in with Atum.

After the Transitions workshop, I sign up for his two-year program, The Art of Spiritual Guidance. I am keenly aware that this period ought to cover Holly's passing and my moving on. This will be an act of continuation for me, a bridge to my unlived life. Eighteen of us will meet with Atum for two workshops at Hollyhock, plus eight weekends in Vancouver. I can only imagine how close we'll become.

When I fly up from California for our first meeting in Vancouver, I'm carrying one of my anti-seizure medications with me, but not the one that could get me in trouble at customs. So when I leave the airport I set out to find some of that storied British Columbia bud.

I take the Canada Line train downtown and walk along Hastings Street to the New Amsterdam Café. I've read about this place online, and sure enough the tables are filled with young people drinking lattes and smoothies, eating grilled-cheese sandwiches (you can order The Cheech or The Chong), and blazing so much reefer they've got smoke shooting out of their ears.

One wall is lined with merchandise. Bongs. Bubblers. Glass and wooden pipes. One-hitters. Vaporizers. Vaping pens. Grinders. Scales. Scentless vacuum jars. Hidey cans. Marijuana-themed underpants.

I ask a man behind the counter: "If dope is against the law, why does the city allow this place to exist?"

"It's not legal," he says. "It's tolerated."

A customer chips in, "Just like prostitution."

The clerk says the café is determined to be a good neighbor. On weekdays, only vaping is allowed on the premises—"so smoke doesn't drift up to the offices above us." After 5 p.m. and on weekends, customers can light up.

It is plain, however, that I won't be able to fulfill my own mission. Prominent signs on the walls proclaim:

You Cannot Buy Cannabis Here. Don't Ask.

I wander next door to the storefront Marijuana Party: Cannabis Culture Headquarters. Here I can buy marijuana magazines and cookbooks and board games and self-testing kits. I can buy a shoulder bag for carrying a water pipe the size of a didgeridoo. But still no marijuana.

According to Yelp, there used to be some bikers living upstairs who would sell you a bag. Now the second floor is a marijuana museum that's closed for the day. The third floor is another quasi-legal smoking den with bongs for rent, clusters of beat-up couches, a pool table, a pinball machine, a couple of cats, portraits on the walls of Haile Selassie, Bob Marley and Marcus Garvey, and a huge monitor streaming live video from the house's own channel, pot.tv.

Yet no pot itself. On the walls are the same don't-ask-we-won't-tell signs.

The two hipsters behind the counter are sucking on each their own joints. It's like you aren't just allowed to smoke in here—you have to. I wonder how I can pose the forbidden question. I venture to the older one, "Can I at least ask you where I *can* ask that question?"

"Not here," he reminds me. "But you're in the right neighborhood."

Fair enough. I go out and loiter on the sidewalk. No one solicits me. Then I spot three teen-agers toking in a park across the street. They're sitting in the shadow of a war memorial inscribed: IT IS NOTHING TO YOU. I saunter up to them. I've come to realize that my advanced age gives me a cachet among young stoners.

I ask them, "So where can an old doper from the States score a little weed around here?"

One kid points down a busy street. "See that ATM?" he says. "Stand there, and a guy with a hat will come by."

"Okay. Thanks."

"It's real good, too!"

"Dynamite!" I cheer, like I'm one of them.

The ATM is in front of a historic youth hostel. I plant myself squarely in front of it. No one approaches. I should have asked: What kind of hat should I look for? Then I see a paunchy guy in a ballcap motioning with one hand. *"This way,"* he whispers.

I follow him into an alley. He asks me: Would I like an eighth-ounce for $40? A quarter-ounce? He pulls a bag out of his coat pocket. I undo the plastic zipper and stick my nose in. Next to us, two men are unloading boxes from a truck. My new friend nods to them as if to acknowledge that we're doing business on their turf.

How much do I want to buy? Over the weekend I won't smoke even an eighth of an ounce. But I'll be coming to Vancouver for three more weekends of spiritual blossoming over the coming months. So I buy a quarter-ounce, with a game plan in mind. Next Monday morning, before I head to the airport to fly home, I will locate some place in this busy city to bury my stash where it won't be disturbed by gardeners or dogs or rodents or drenching winter storms.

Why am I drawn to this man Atum?

Because he puts my instincts for self-preservation into a larger, grander context, letting me see that I'm part of a more meaningful, uplifting, universal scheme.

Because he turns shit into gold. He listens to some nebulous idea of mine, then reframes it—gives it just a quarter-turn—to make it sound like I've actually said something wise.

Because his voice is both soothing and authoritative, both suggestive and precise, a voice that's a melody gently rising and falling, a voice that lulls me awake.

Because he remembers every foible I have revealed, and he encourages me to be my boldest, bravest self.

One day he sidles up, puts a hand on my shoulder, and suggests, "Don't ever lose that boyish nature of yours."

I take it to be a commandment.

Another day he talks to us about answering the call to seek spiritual guidance. "The call is an invitation," he says, "not a demand. It's a call into life. It's a call to wholeness. And it's not about your worthiness, because the call can transform you to what it needs."

Here I have to interrupt, to ask about something that has bothered me from the start. I tell him, "I have a question that might get me kicked out of this program."

It's meant to get a laugh, and it does. Atum lifts an eyebrow mischievously. "I can't wait to hear what it is."

"What I want to know," I say, "is this. How can a person think about answering the call if he doesn't even know if he believes in a god? In any god?"

His answer is so simple, so inclusive, so forgiving, so magnanimous. "To believe in a god or a supreme being," he intones, "is merely to believe that there's some power higher than your own ego."

That's all there is to it? "You set the bar so low," I tell him.

I come to my feet and take a small step forward, first with one foot, then the other foot.

"There! I believe!"

An obvious question I could ask myself is: Why do I want to be stoned in this sacred setting, of all places? Isn't there a howling disconnect between a drug-inspired high and an authentic spiritual high?

Maybe. Maybe not.

All of us here—in this workshop, in this world—are looking for some confirmation that we're getting nearer to living in harmony with our deepest drumbeats. What can we trust in this enterprise but our own truest instincts? Because of my boyish energy and my years of sacrifices for Holly and my eagerness now to rejoin the human circus, I have no inclination to be discriminating about where I look for or find enlightenment. As a friend in Colorado says, "I want everything all the time starting now." I want to seek the guidance of sages and poets, and in the short run I want to repeatedly brighten the inner walls of my skull by whatever nontoxic means I have at my disposal.

My rationale for holding onto this habit is that it has worked for me since dinosaurs roamed the earth. My stoned self is who I want to be: my best self. So the only question left as we wrap up another glowing weekend in Vancouver is: Where am I going to bury my medicine?

On my return visits I'll be staying in two different bed-and-breakfasts. So I split the remaining herbs into two emptied-out pill bottles.

First, in the Kitsilano neighborhood, I snoop around the side yard of Simone's B&B, where I've just finished my eggs benedict. At the corner of the house is a flowerbed that looks promisingly untended. I poke two fingers into the dirt. Good: all soft and leafy. I bury the Vitamin B-12 bottle several inches under. Then I stand back and stare at the gravesite to fix its location in my memory, because occasionally I forget things.

I hide the other bottle in the fancier Shaughnessy neighborhood, in a lightly trafficked alley near the other B&B, up against a fence. I mark the spot with a scrap of orange plastic from some kid's trashed Halloween basket.

Then I fly home to California to look after Holly. But the following month, and the month after that, and the month after that I will have the privilege of returning to Vancouver to reawaken the spirit within me, and to dig into the earth for buried pleasures.

Many weeks later, I get an e-mail from Simone, my B&B hostess in Kitsilano. It says:

"Hey Tom. I just wanted to let you know that the other day we pulled out a plant from the garden on the side of the house and lo and behold we found your stash. It is in our kitchen beside the microwave. When you get here next weekend, just ask Coreen to pass it along to you."

Vancouver is such a hospitable city.

Ghosts

2014
Make Me an Angel

Holly doesn't return to our ghost town in the summers anymore. The three-day drive from California is too much. At high altitude she can't get enough oxygen. She has lost interest in her old friends. She seems to have very little room left in her consciousness for this place she called home for half of her life. She's a ghost now herself.

To me, it's still home, and I come back when I can get away, for two or three weeks at a stretch.

On the eve of the Fourth of July I fly into Denver for the summer's first visit. I rent a car, and when I reach Boulder I can't resist stopping at one of the marijuana stores which have opened in the six months since Colorado became the first state to go whole-hog legal.

I try the outlet called Terrapin Station, because I'm familiar with the location. It's the old Dunkin' Donuts shop on Canyon and Folsom. At 5 o'clock on the opening night of a holiday weekend, the parking lot is full. I see through the window that the reception area is jammed. I have to park two blocks away and start hiking.

Doughnuts never sold like this.

We have come so far from the days when buying dope was a subversive act, an adventure. That used to be part of the intrigue: the knowing that you were breaking the law.

I first got turned on by Barry Shapiro, who worked with me on the *Daily Collegian* newspaper at Wayne State University in Detroit. One day he slipped me a joint and said I'd know it was taking effect when my legs felt heavy. I was 19, still living with my parents. That night I went up to my bedroom, its walls papered with 1951 baseball cards. I smoked the joint and sat there for a long time trying to feel how my legs felt. Then I went to bed.

Ten years later, when I discovered that pot wasn't about a heaviness in the limbs but a lightness in the belfry, I bought it from friends who were turning me on. Then I graduated to having my own dealer.

I liked the racy image, going to a dealer, even if the transaction was usually stilted and predictable. It was always a guy, never a woman. I'd slouch over to his house, and we'd sit in the living room and exchange small talk. Then he'd disappear into a back room and bring out a baggie and drop it on the coffeetable. He had just this one kind, take it or leave it. I'd open the bag and sniff and say something like, "Real skunky!", as if I knew what primo grass ought to smell like. We both had to pretend that I was weighing whether to buy it or not.

He'd roll a joint. We'd pass it.

He'd ask, "So waddya think?"

Holding the smoke in, my jowls ballooned out, I'd grin like a moron and nod my head in vigorous approval.

But, hell, I didn't know how good the stuff was. How high I got had more to do with my readiness of mind and the comfort of my setting than it did the quality of the weed. This was a business meeting, a formality. I wouldn't know if it was any good until I tried it at home. And even then all of the strains lifted me to about the same elevation.

One long-time supplier, Jax, drove a road-grader for the county. He was eccentric, like most mountain people. He was a rock hound and was self-publishing a book about it. When I dropped by his cabin, his wife and kids were there, along with his pet ocelot, who I figured could have eaten any one of us. At other times, if I was running low on smoke I waved Jax down when I saw his snowplow coming.

Now I usually buy from Gabor, a soft-spoken recluse from Hungary. He's a generous host—serves his customers tea and sweets from his homeland. He grows his bud in the back yard and takes pride in its organic purity. His wife has a degenerative disease whose symptoms are alleviated by smoking. Sitting down with the two of them to sample the latest crop is a real commitment—a nonstop merry-go-round of joints and pipes and bongs and Volcano bags and vaping pens. Gabor and Jenny are marvels. They smoke from the first light of day until their heads hit the pillow again.

Now that marijuana is legal, what will happen to these lovable black-marketeers?

They can undercut the dispensaries, in part because they don't charge taxes. But Gabor tells me his business has fallen off by half, and the future looks even worse. The spread of legalization could lead to super-efficient corporate farms which bring prices down so low the little guys could never compete. That's how America works.

I walk into Dunkin' Donuts—into Terrapin Station—and a uniformed guard checks my driver's license. What is he looking for? Is there an upper age limit?

I take a number from a machine: 991.

The message board says: *Now being served...968.*

I take a seat in the waiting room.

The patrons are men and women, young and old, shaggy and trimmed. One by one, they enter the sales sanctum. My number comes up after twenty minutes. I go in to see well-dressed clerks standing behind glass display cases like they're selling diamonds. I ask a girl: "What do you have that'll give me a good creative inspirational head-rush?"

It's refreshingly above-board—to not have to pretend that it's some physical pain I'm here to cure, but to admit that the ache is existential.

She informs me that the pricier strains are sold out. She recommends one I'm not familiar with. Does she know what she's talking about? That's always the question with dealers, legal or illegal.

You have to have faith. Remember this: If you expect it will get you high, you're already halfway there.

The flowering of legalization and commercialization going on across the country takes me back 37 years to 1977, when I was living in the attic at NORML. That was the last high point in the campaign to gain legal acceptance for marijuana. What a year it was, 1977—so ahead of its time that a celebrity lobbyist they called Mr. Marijuana was drafting presidential speeches.

Since 1969 the Gallup Poll has been asking Americans: "Do you think the use of marijuana should be made legal, or not?" In 1977 a record-high 28% said "yes." Then the figure leveled out until the century's end, when it was still only 31%. By 2013, amazingly, it had shot up to 58%.

In 1977, it looked like legalization was right around the corner. It looks even more like that today, with state barriers falling one by one. But you never know when something could upset the apple cart—a TMZ clip of cops getting stoned in Denver...a video of a toddler standing next to a Christmas tree licking a THC-doped candy cane.

After buying a quarter-ounce of Terrapin Station's second-best and stopping to get groceries, I drive up to our little town. It's 7 in the evening, the summer sun still riding high over the Continental Divide. The last two miles take me along the treacherous Shelf Road, which drops off a thousand feet into Lefthand Canyon. Then the road noses down, and our town comes into view: the white steeple of the schoolhouse, the false-fronted General Store, the shuttered log hotel.

Our cabin is perched on a west-facing ridge looking down over the town and out to the peaks. I gun the rental car up the steep driveway and park at the bottom of the stone steps which lead to the house. I will never forget that Holly built these steps herself, boulder by boulder.

I walk into the door for the first time in nine months, and the phone is ringing. It's my friends Rebecca and Janos. Can I come over for dinner?

How did I get so popular? My friends hold me in absurdly high regard because of how I've stuck it out with Holly. I know what a far cry I am from being a saint. I get annoyed with her for things she can't control. I can sound aggrieved or exhausted. I assure my married friends, "I'm only doing what you'd do in the same situation."

People like being around me, I think, because when I'm away from my caregiving gig I'm a guy who has broken out of jail. I come alive in a high-voltage way that's possible only for someone who, from one decade to the next, has had to get by as a cooped-up, scaled-down, burned-out, shut-in version of his true self. When I'm in Colorado or British Columbia, I love everybody, and everybody (or so I pretend) loves me. And marijuana just amps up this electrification.

Many of my old mountain friends, in their sixties and seventies, have cut back on smoking grass. Some find it hard on their lungs, or too strong compared with the dope of yesteryear. Some report feeling slow and draggy the day after. Some have just outgrown it. Not me.

The Fourth of July in our town begins with a pancake breakfast in the yard of the two-room schoolhouse. It's a benefit for the volunteer fire department, and I run into people I haven't seen for ages. Some of my friends are busy flipping pancakes—Everett and Madeline, Max the heavy-equipment guy, the whole firehouse crew.

At noon there's a makeshift parade down the dusty main street. Fire engines with their sirens wailing and kids sitting on top...teenagers riding horses...antique pickups and jalopies...water-cannon fights. House parties all over town. Bear and Poppy welcome whoever drops by. Devin and Mark are having a jam on their front porch. A Cajun band is playing in the side yard of the saloon.

On the night of the Fourth, half a dozen of us pile into a car and pass around a doob and drive up to another old mining camp—a more outlaw town, 1000 feet higher and ten miles farther from the bright lights. We are going to join a spectacle they have here every Fourth of July.

The War Zone, it's called.

At the edge of their town, we park at Jax's house. He drives us in his open-air Jeep toward the baseball field, which is laid out on top of the old town dump. I used to play here on Sundays when we had home-and-home softball games. I remember how their catcher described his team: "The infield's on probation and the outfield's on parole."

Jax eases us down a rutted road through the woods, the air heavy with smoke. We emerge onto the field, and it's a freak show, a battle-ground—gangs of locals standing back and shooting fireworks at each other. Bottle rockets and buzz-bombs volleying across the field, hiss-ing, screaming, whistling, skittering along the ground, arching over our heads, exploding in front of us, reverberating through our chests, showering us with sparks.

The skies overhead are ablaze with the town's official fireworks show. Each aerial concussion illuminates our hell-on-earth below.

And the rocket's red glare,
The bombs bursting in air...

We're wearing safety glasses. We're bundled up in blast suits. We're having way too much fun to be afraid.

Gave proof through the night
That our flag was still there...

Heavy metal pumping out. The night stinking of burnt sulfur and ganja. Lunatics dancing for attention like targets in a shooting gal-lery, their herky-jerky movements silhouetted against the white-hot bombardments.

A young woman strolls into the fray leading a toddler by one hand and holding an explosive in the other.

O'er the land of the free,
And the home of the brave!

Forty years have gone by since Holly and I answered John Denver's call and moved to the Rockies. Since then, not much about our town has changed. The population still hovers around 100. The roads are still dirt. The textures are rugged—of logs and chinking and rough-sawn planking. We still have one store, one restaurant, no churches and no clipped lawns. Our yard sculptures are junked trucks and potbelly stoves. Our Indian sweat lodges have given way to hot tubs. Most people have plumbing instead of outhouses. But the hippies never did leave. We own the joint now.

In the days following the Fourth, there are more town parties, and they usually end up with a knot of musicians gathering on somebody's porch.

Take a load off, Fanny, Take a load for free...

A bunch of guitars, a banjo, a harmonica, a keyboard. Jax and Becky. Larry and Bear. The new guy Billy Shaddox.

Gonna take a freight train, down at the station...

Mary Russell wailing like Janice Joplin. Old Bill Atkinson shouting out the hollers of his native Oklahoma. Young Brandy, a granddaughter of 1960s settlers, working the fiddle.

Can't you see, can't you see,
What that woman, she been doin' to me?

I think about Holly. She'd like being here with our friends. Or the old Holly would have.

When I come back here every summer, people ask, "How's Holly?" I shake my head and say, "Well, she's hangin' in there." Or, "She's a trooper, you know." This year they aren't asking as much. They know what the score is.

They sing John Prine's old lament about aging:

Make me an angel that flies from Montgomery...

I stand on Larry's porch gazing out over the town meadow and the blackened pine trees on the hillside above. Four years ago, while Holly and I were away, the most damaging forest fire in Colorado's history nearly wiped us off the map. It came up to the edge of town before slurry bombers and ground troops (including some of our most prominent dopers and drinkers) rallied to beat it back.

To believe in this livin' is just a hard way to go

Damn, I've got tears in my eyes again.

2014
Old Stoners

Everett is our ghost town's cookie master. He grows the active ingredient. He bakes the cookies and sells them for two bucks apiece. He raises his prices only at the autumn bake sale, when the money goes to charity.

Many of Everett's customers are older women who find smoking too harsh now and who prefer the subtler, longer-lasting invigorations of eating marijuana. Me, I like the breathtaking lift that I get from firing up, which is what Everett and I do together as the two leading stoners in our circle. But anyone who hangs out with our crowd for very long will hear the admission: "I just ate one of Everett's cookies." As if to apologize for any excessive candor or lapses in etiquette over the next four or five hours.

Everett and Madeline live on top of the tallest ridge around, in a hand-built cabin near the end of a bad road. They have glorious views of both the divide and the Great Plains, but not much in the way of public services. At first they lit their place with kerosene and candles and crapped in an outhouse. When they got married in 1981 they put up solar panels to bring in electricity. In '97 they built a rain-catchment system. Presto: running water.

My house is lower down on the same ridge, a ten-minute walk away. I'm back in town again for two weeks, for the frivolities surrounding Labor Day. More parties. A poetry reading. More community. More music. More happy tears.

One day I hike up to visit Everett and see how his garden is growing. He walks me around to inspect his six plants. He grows them in five-gallon buckets to keep voles from eating the roots and to make them portable, so they can be moved inside if there's an early frost. A month before harvest time, the plants are shoulder high. We examine their pistils with a magnifying lens. "See those little clear crystal balls?" he says. "That's the THC."

These six plants will take care of his desires for a year. The buds are for smoking. The leaves and stems are for making cookies, which is simple enough. "I take it and put it in a pressure cooker, and I add water, then a couple sticks of butter. The THC goes to oil easier than it goes to water. So that's the butter I use to make the cookies.

"This right here," he says, pointing to the plants, "is why they'll never get a handle on commercializing it—because anybody can do it. They're never going to be able to regulate it like they do cigarettes and alcohol."

Everett is six-foot-three, with a wizardly gray beard. He's a Long Islander by birth: modest, laconic. "I keep my garden low-key," he tells me. "I don't want to be ripped off. I'm not trying to do anything but get some pot and smoke it and give it away and make cookies. It's fun. I enjoy growing pot. I enjoy the plants developing."

We go inside and sit down. Madeline is home, along with their two kittens, Willie and Waylon.

Everett informs her, "We'll have a little toke to help Tommy in his research."

It's last year's crop, as pungent as ever.

Madeline volunteers her opinion: "I feel like pot really improved my life because I grew up in this alcoholic family, and I felt like I had to try to control everything because it could go crazy on me at any time. So you're always watching out and you're trying to be careful..."

"You try not to upset people," says Everett.

She nods. "You don't upset people. You want to keep under the radar. Even after I moved to the mountains, everything had to be just so. And pot just lets you relax with that stuff. You realize the world is going to go on. It's not counting on me to control it. I can get a little deeper into life and a little less into straightening everything and cleaning and organizing and bossing."

Everett testifies, "I don't know if I would have survived without smoking pot, because of my father's and brother's predilections. I would have drunk too much. I would have been destroyed by alcohol or been killed in a car. Instead of getting drunk, it's just more pleasant to be high. It's better to be stoned than loaded."

Madeline remembers the first time she tried it: "My husband John hands me a lid off a shoe box and says, 'Take out the seeds and stems.' I say, 'What is this?' And he says, 'That's marijuana. Want to try it?' So I'm sitting there smoking, and I'm thinking nothing's happening, and then I realize that I can make myself bigger or littler. Or I can stay the same size and make the room bigger or littler. And John says, 'I think you've had enough.'"

Everett remembers his introduction: "It felt like a little lightning bolt went up my spine and into my brain, and I said, 'This is cool.' And I wanted to do it again.

"On a lot of levels for me," he understands, "it's an antidepressant. If I smoke pot I get more energized. I get more interested in things, and I want to do things."

What else can he say?

"I'm a pothead. It works for me."

The next day, with my time in Colorado ticking down, I drive to the town cemetery with Everett and Madeline and our friend Sharon, a psychologist who is one of Everett's veteran cookie subscribers. Usually I think of graveyards as being on flat ground. But there is no such land around here. Our cemetery was built, in 1866, on an upward-sloping hillside along a back road. It is enclosed by a half-fallen wire fence. The lower section, near the road, is clustered with aspens and pines. The higher ground is more open, with vistas out over the plains.

Today is a foggy, clammy day. It was foggy, we remember, when we helped Ron and Bonnie bury their infant son Jonathan here in 1977, on the day after Easter. It was foggy when we buried Gabor's first wife, Victoria, here.

Madeline and Everett have been married for more than thirty years. Sharon has been a widow for fifteen years. I am soon to be widowed. Yet our missions here are the same. We are looking for places to bury our ashes, and to celebrate in chiseled stone our presence upon this cherished piece of earth. The plots are only $100, and it's time. I want one for Holly, and one for myself.

The first graves we come to are the older graves, from the 1800s, and what a sad story they tell. Here lies Alice Hastings, who died at 16. Here is Maude Hastings, also 16. Florence Hastings, 13. Eileen Coughlin, 21. Margaret Coughlin, 10. John Coughlin, 3. Six children from only two families. Another stone says: "Our baby. Died Aug. 12, 1888. Age 27 days."

We walk farther up the hill, looking for newer, more familiar names. But we can find hardly any of them, and I feel a loneliness, a hollowed-outness, sweeping over me. The day is cool. The aspens are already turning yellow. I don't want to bury Holly among strangers. I don't want to spend eternity with strangers myself. I look around me. Where are all of our friends?

Well, duhhh. We're not dead yet! Not quite.

Holly will be our pioneer.

We grave-seekers are accompanied by our neighbor Dale, who is the long-time chairman (and I believe the only member) of the town's cemetery committee. While my best local friends are smart-ass college graduates from distant parts of the country, Dale is a true local. His people go back to the mining days. He is a good carpenter who may have fallen off the wagon a few times earlier in life. But when that fire swept down upon our town, Dale was one of those do-or-die characters (in part the saloonkeepers and their oldest customers) who defied the evacuation order and stayed behind to fight it.

Dale is carrying a sheaf of papers which purport to show, approximately, where people have been buried here, or where they want to be buried. He muses that in the old days he had to dig the graves for the caskets by hand. Now it's easier. He uses a post-hole digger for the urns.

The four of us wander around, lost in the seriousness, or the meaninglessness, of this quest. I wonder: What if Dale dies first? Who will take care of our final needs?

Madeline declares, "I want to be buried where I can see our house!"

I needle, "You going to have a periscope down there?"

She and Everett find the spot in the upper part of the graveyard where, after the fire, they planted two trees—a spruce and an aspen. Yes, Madeline confirms, this is where they want to be: between the two saplings. Dale marks it in his ledger.

Sharon tells Madeline and Everett to lie down on their backs, next to each other, on top of their gravesites. She asks them to close their eyes. Then she pulls out her cell phone and takes their picture, to make it official.

Sharon wants her own plot to be lower down, nearer to the entrance, so that visitors won't miss her headstone. The stone will be a joke, a takeoff on the sign she put up on the road coming into town—the sign that announces:

Founded   1859
Elevation   8463
Population   118
TOTAL   10,440

Her headstone will say (depending on when she dies):

Born   1937
Husbands 1
Children 3
Died   2020
TOTAL 3,961

Even in death, this woman will get laughs.

The site she selects is in a lush aspen grove, with tall grasses all around. It's not far from the resting place of that memorable reprobate, Uncle Fred. Nearby is a wooden bench where Sharon's many acquaintances can sit and contemplate what a caring yet carefree soul she was.

I take her phone and tell her, "Lie down and play dead." I have to add, "Close your eyes. And stop laughing."

I take her picture. Dale marks it in his ledger.

I, too, feel drawn toward this shady patch of grassy ground. Holly loved aspens. She wrote poems about them: about how in the autumn the leaves fluttered in the breeze like gold coins. She painted aspens. I think that if she had a chance to stand here with us, she would like this restful place. I will describe it to her as best I can.

I move over three giant steps from Sharon's sacred (or not so sacred) site. Don't want to cramp her style.

I hand Dale the 200 bucks. I hand Sharon the phone.

I lie on my back and stretch out my arms, to make room for two. I close my eyes. "Okay, we're going in here."

Our mortuary detail is over. The sun is coming out. We drive to the town's bocce court to roll a few balls.

When we were younger, we played softball. We called our field Rock Stadium, for the granite outcroppings which gave the game its zany pinball effect. Everett was the shortstop; I played third; Dale was at second, Sharon at first; Madeline pitched. Often there'd be a keg of beer from someone's party the night before. On summer evenings we played volleyball in Kirby's Field. Every Thanksgiving and Christmas we had a touch football game that was called the Roach Bowl, after the form of halftime entertainment.

Now it's bocce—that Italian bowling game which favors finesse over strength, thus erasing the gender gap and the age gap all at once. In the late 1990s a neighbor, Karl, built a court in his yard, and a tournament was held every July. We could practice there any time, and this became a popular way for us underemployed misfits to socialize.

Early this year, Karl and his wife sold their house and moved down to Boulder. The new owner promised to let the bocce tournaments continue. But then his roommate, a high-school classmate and small-time marijuana dealer, got murdered out on the plains in a deal gone wrong. Rumors spread that Karl's place was now a grow house. Hell, all we cared about was that our bocce court was going to ruin.

A movement welled up to build a court of our own, a loitering ground that couldn't ever be taken away. Charles and Torkin donated the land on Kirby's Field. My bocce partner Bear, a retired engineering professor, took charge. He sent around e-mails asking for $1,500 to cover the costs. He got $1,800 pledged in the first 24 hours.

Bear and I drove out to Longmont to pick up the 6-by-6 timbers that would define the court. Max rumbled in on his backhoe to scrape the sod off of a 120-foot-long swath of dirt. Work parties convened. Gravel was trucked in and raked smooth. Max brought in the finishing material—a small-grained sandy mixture that, in the rock business, went by the name of "crusher fines." Finally, we hauled a 300-pound roller up and down and up and down the court to make the fines even finer.

In two months, on Labor Day weekend, we held our first tournament—a rollicking display of small-town fellowship. Sixteen two-person teams. Spectators lining both sides of the court. Pop-up awnings for shade; tables freighted with potluck dishes; coolers of beer; Everett's cookies. Some of the gals wanted just a quarter-cookie buzz. Others went for a half. The tournament started at 8 in the morning and lasted until 4 in the afternoon, after which it seemed only appropriate to go over to Bear's and plop into the hot tub.

Now, a few days later, we four senior slackers, having reserved our plots in the cemetery, are back in the game again, back on the court, rolling balls.

Sharon and I don't usually team up together. But we're both from Detroit. If there's one thing you learn there, it's how to bowl. Madeline and Everett are a hard pair to beat. They're the four-time town champions. She always rolls first for them; the big guy rolls clean-up.

Our new court isn't as smooth as our old one. There are little saddles and ruts. A ball can tail off this way or that without explanation. At the end of its journey it might wobble like a drunk. The angles for bank shots are less reliable. But that's okay. There is not one thing about our town that is straight or on the level.

One after the other, we roll the balls. Green balls for them, red balls for us. Two balls per person. Eight balls to a round—or to a *giro*, as we say in Italian.

Then we saunter down to see who's the closest.

Madeline eyes the formation of balls. "One green," she rules.

"One green," Sharon concurs.

I rack it up on the scoreboard. "One green."

The rhythms are reassuring. We could be playing shuffleboard. This could be 1956. We're the ghosts of our grandparents. We should pipe in Sinatra.

We kick the balls behind the foul line and get ready to roll them back the other way.

I have a question for Everett. I know what the answer is going to be. It's less of a question than a suggestion, a nudge.

I turn to him: "You bring a joint?"

Gratefully, he reaches into his pack.

"IT'S DE RIGEUR!" he exults.

2015
The Clean Plate Award

Holly's caregiver wakes her up from her nap at 5:30. Regina helps her into the bathroom, then into the sitting room to get comfortable on the couch. She brings her a plate of fruit—strawberries, raspberries, blueberries.

This is often Holly's liveliest, most responsive time of the day. She is well-rested, and she has always loved to eat. It's one of the few pleasures she has managed to hold onto. She will sit on the couch and pick up those berries one by one by one and feed herself patiently and contentedly throughout the evening news and beyond.

She is extremely good at focusing on what's directly in front of her. Her awareness keeps narrowing to the bare essentials. She pays scant attention to the past or the future. She has realized her spiritual ambition, it seems: to live in the here and now. Congratulations, sweetheart.

I come into the room and see her leaning intently over her fruit, and it touches me, how this small offering is enough to brighten her countenance.

"Hi, honey!" I call.

"Hi, Tom!"

Regina and I look at each other, startled to hear her speak up so loudly and clearly.

I kiss her on the forehead, and she gives me that game-girl smile which can sometimes break my heart. She looks so fragile and vulnerable, but at the same time resolute: her inner Holly struggling to burst through this withered shell.

She points to her plate and says something. I lean closer to hear. I can't understand every word, but she's talking about the blueberries.

She seems to be remarking that they look like beads.

I try to clarify: "Like beads from a necklace?"

She nods.

"You're right!" I cheerlead. "Or from a bracelet!" It's good to hear her string together a sentence or two. "*Exactly* like beads!" I belabor.

The conversation appears to have run its course. I start moving away to do something else. But she has more to say.

I lean down again.

She asks, with a child-like sense of trust in her voice, "Do you think they're safe to eat?"

Oh. I see. She suspects that they really are beads.

I rest a hand on her bony shoulder. "I'm sure they'll be fine, honey."

She looks up at me. That game smile. She seems to believe me, that it will be all right.

So many times I wonder: What is she thinking?

I never know which Holly I'm going to see. Sometimes her face is a blank, her eyes not tracking, her jaw dropped open. When I walk her to the bathroom, she'll turn the wrong way, forgetting where the bathroom is, or what we're doing. At other times, her face is lit up with amusement, and it's plain that more is going on upstairs than she can express. She's able to follow stories. Out of the blue she'll rekindle a long-expired conversation. Her words are few, but her vocabulary is rich. If I prompt her, she can recollect minor details of long-ago trips.

I struggle to imagine what it would be like to be in her slippers. Once so proudly independent, she now has virtually no control over her days. Once so brimming with initiative, she is now led around by the hand or pushed from behind, from the bed to the bathroom to the dining room and back again, following other people's priorities.

We speak to her gently but insistently:

"Let's have breakfast now, okay?"

"It's time for your smoothie."

"Do you want to lie down, Holly?"

"It's time to get up."

Sometimes she resists. She leans back against being pushed—puts on the brakes. She grabs onto a doorjamb to assert herself, to be listened to, even if she can't get the words out. For a caregiver it's frustrating. For Holly it's one defeat after another, to be consigned to this never-ending helplessness, this breakdown of self.

But I want to give her the credit she is due. Because over twenty years of decline she has hardly ever complained about her lot. She has never asked: "Why me?" Never. I have wondered whether this is because of her decades of contemplative work, or because the part of her brain having to do with regret or self-pity is burned out. Maybe it's a blessed marriage of the two.

She has rarely complained about pain, either, except for those years of agonies from drug withdrawal. Again I have to guess. Has her pain center gone offline? Or has she brought this good fortune upon herself?

I can't ignore the positive aspects of how she has turned out. In the old days she fretted about never having enough time to accomplish everything she wanted to do. Now time is not the enemy. It's on her side. She can relax. She doesn't have to prove her smarts by getting another book published; doesn't have to prove her goodness by counseling another troubled child; doesn't have to play Ms. Natural and study nutritional labels; doesn't have to be the prettiest girl in the room; doesn't have to be perfect.

Marijuana remains an ally for her. Smoking it makes her cough, so I've tried giving her five or six drops of cannabis oil following her afternoon nap. For the first couple of hours, the medicine fails to arouse her. Oil on the tongue doesn't deliver the on-demand high that smoking provides. But later in the evening, toward bedtime, I'll catch her laughing for no apparent reason, and when we tuck her in she is pleasantly aglow.

Sweet dreams, sweetheart.

The clock is winding down. I've stopped taking her in for medical examinations. No more appointments with the dermatologist to search for pre-cancers. No more check-ups at the gynecologist. No more dental maintenance. These are crummy decisions to make. I am betting on her dying.

I'm putting off a hernia-repair operation for myself because for a month afterward I wouldn't be able to lift anything heavy, such as a wife. I'm betting that pretty soon I will no longer have that burden. I'm putting off a mold-removal project in my upstairs bedroom because I'd have nowhere to sleep. The downstairs is a hospice unit now. I'm betting that a bed will open up.

During our forty years together, I have long since gotten used to waiting for Holly. In the old days my role was to stand by the front door waiting to go to a party while she tried on fifty different combinations of skirts and sweaters and scarves. As the Parkinson's made all of her movements and deliberations slower and slower, those waits became longer and longer and longer.

Now I'm not waiting for her to join me anymore. I'm waiting for her to leave me.

Holly's nurse Dianne, an LVN with a dim regard for Western medicine, has worked in the hospice field for decades. Two years ago I asked her, "Can you give me a ballpark guess about how long she might last?"

She told me, "In terms of her life force, I would say one or two years. But some people have the will power or the stubbornness to go on longer."

I said, "I don't know if Holly fits that description. I've never seen anybody die slowly. My people die in an instant. Heart attacks. A bullet to the head. You're a hospice nurse. Wouldn't you be the best judge?"

"No," she said. "You would."

It perplexed me: the answer. I was well-acquainted with Holly's inherited fears about her health. But in the face of this disease I had mainly been impressed by her courage. Did she have the will power to keep keeping on? Was she stubborn enough?

Now I'm surprised at how blind I was. Of course she has the mettle. Look at the strength of will it took in the '70s for her to leave her husband, break up her family and renounce every advantage her parents ever gave her in order to create a more fulfilling and empowering and novel destiny for herself. That same strength, or some image of it, still dwells within her.

She weighs 90 pounds, down from 125. Still, look at how diligently she attends to eating her meals, like some Zen priestess—bowing her head, spooning each bite slowly and shakily but relentlessly in the direction of her mouth, not letting me take over the spoon, not lifting her head, not losing her focus no matter how long it takes—thirty minutes, forty minutes—until the practice is complete.

When her son Scott visits us, he loves to call out at the end of a meal: "Mom wins the Clean Plate Award!"

I have assembled such a loving crew of women to take care of her that maybe it's not in our best interests. My wish is for her to die sooner rather than later, to die in peace rather than misery. Yet here she is with a game-winning support network—a parade of hired girlfriends who come in to cook good meals and help her play dress-up and comb her hair and read to her and cater to her every whim.

All of us agree that our aim is to improve her quality of life, not merely to prolong it. But how can we know which end we are serving? All we can do is to serve.

I ask myself: If I were in Holly's position, would I want to keep on living? The answer I get is: Who wouldn't want to go on being treated like a princess? Especially if you were born a princess.

I catch myself yearning for this struggle to be over, longing to be released. But in the 1970s we had a maxim: "Don't push the river." Why should I be impatient to begin an uncertain future when this experience right now is so meaningful, so primal? I think that my helpers and I will look back upon this long good-bye with Holly as a time of inspiration and intimacy and camaraderie. This doesn't feel like a death watch, but more like a witnessing of how precious life can be, for Holly to hold onto it so dearly.

When she does finally surrender, I expect to be left with a smorgasbord of reactions—incredulity, desolation, relief. I used to assure my friends: "I've already done my grieving." But that was premature. Yes, I've mourned the loss of my enthusiastic sidekick in adventure. But how can I know how I'll feel when she vanishes altogether?

She will go from being the center of my universe to a mere apparition. My consuming mission for all these years, the mission which has remodeled my character, will be over.

How will I replace that?

Volunteer work? Disaster relief?

Pilgrimages abroad with Atum? Doing a book with him?

I prepare for my unlived life by weighing the options. But all I really know is that suddenly one day I am going to have no one to check in on, no one to listen for, no helpers coming over, no one to talk to, no rhythms to the day, no schedules, no routines, no diapers to buy, no rubber gloves, no pills to count out, no nothing.

What will it be like to wake up that first morning without her being here, without her being anywhere? Will I check her bed, to make sure?

I'll start the day like it's any other day. Making coffee. Retrieving the *New York Times* from the bushes. Sitting by the window reading it. Getting used to this big house, this awesome silence. I'll save the sports section for last, as usual. Then I'll check my watch.

Only 8:15?

Now what? A walk?

With no obligations, I'll be free to walk all day. No one will notice when I come back. No one will care. No one will know if I never come back. I won't have anybody to look after, and I won't have anybody looking after me.

A level playing field. A new game.

2016
Her Last Words?

Dying isn't part of her repertoire. It has no place in her self-image. I keep thinking that the next holiday season is going to be her last one, and she keeps proving me wrong. Now another New Year's has come and gone.

Her limbs are skeletal. She's in a wheelchair. Her feet are swollen from poor circulation. Her breathing is shallow and congested. Her digestive system is shot. She sleeps eighteen hours a day. Trying to talk with her is a crapshoot. Still, this creature of spirit rallies on.

Is it virtuous, or admirable, or brave, to continue living even after the joys of living are gone?

Or maybe they're not gone. It touches my heart when I see her face light up with affection at the sight of a caregiver arriving to start her shift. Holly wants to keep this merry-go-round going. Is it ours to question why?

Several evenings a week, I leave her with a helper and go out to dinner by myself. This serves two purposes. It gets me out of the house, away from the drama, away from the boredom. And it throws open the door to inspiration.

The routine rarely changes. I go to a friendly (but not too friendly) bar-and-grill, and select a stool where I have plenty of elbow room and the mute companionship of a sports screen nearby. I relish the kind of solitude, the anonymity, that comes from being alone in a crowd. I order a glass of merlot and unfold a few pages of some story I'm working on. Then I drift out to the parking lot and gaze at the stars and take two healthy hits on a pocket pipe.

Back inside, I taste the wine, and it magnifies the sense of lyrical disorientation. My happy old head is chock-full of yippee, teeming with brash expectations and unfounded optimism and big ideas raining down from above. Now, when I pick up those pages of writing, I look at the words with new eyes, as if I've hardly seen them before.

Recently I gave up marijuana for five days in advance of the surgery that I'd been putting off. I was pleased to see that I enjoyed those five days, even if my world wasn't as sparkly or my work as creative. During the dope-fast, I had my usual evenings out. I followed the same routines—the welcoming barroom, the pages of writing, the merlot— except for one part: I didn't sneak out to the parking lot to perfume the night air. And those evenings went well enough. I watched some games on ESPN. But where were the fresh eyes?, the jazzy ideas?

Now the surgery is over. I'm back to my old tricks.

On a Friday night, I return from dinner at 8 o'clock to find Holly sitting on her bedside commode. Plainly, she is distressed, but she can't manage to say what's wrong. Her caregiver Janet and I try to comfort her, and after a while we get her up and into bed. We lie her carefully on her side to protect the pressure sore on her tailbone from further aggravation. She's slipping toward sleep.

I tiptoe away, heading for the refuge of my own room upstairs. Then Janet calls: "Holly's asking for you." So I kneel next to her bed, and she attempts to say something. Her voice is so faint and indistinct, and yet so insistent, as if this is something extremely important. She's frustrated that she can't make herself understood. I strain to pick up even a hint of the subject matter.

Is she trying to say good-bye? I lean closer, my head against hers. What if these are the last words she ever utters? Will I always have to wonder what she said?

I soothe her, in case she needs my permission: "Honey, you are on a journey, and I want you to know that whatever happens with you— whatever—it will be all right for the rest of us. I'll be all right, and so will everybody else. Whatever happens. We'll be okay."

I have voiced such a sentiment before. But maybe she needs to hear it now. Maybe I need to say it now.

Finally, she musters up the wherewithal to speak, to express what's on her mind (her fears?, her regrets?, her hopes?, her gratitude?) at this most tender moment in our unending time together.

She whispers, "We...need...more...butter."

I pat her on the shoulder.

What is there to say?

"I'm going shopping in the morning, honey."

She closes her eyes, reassured.

Acknowledgments

Thank you so much to:

Annie Leibovitz, who generously provided the photograph which graces the front cover;

my publisher Naomi Rosenblatt, for her artist's eye and her steady hand, and for being a dream to work with;

my editor and social-media coach Marla Miller, for her astute editorial judgment and for guiding me through the sticky thickets of publishing and marketing;

Catherine Hiller, author of *Just Say Yes: A Marijuana Memoir*, for blazing the trail;

my friends, my children and my stepchildren, who remain well-springs of joy, comfort and camaraderie.

Author Bio

Born and raised: the streets of Detroit

1959-63: editor, the *Wayne State Daily Collegian*, Detroit

1963-66: copy editor, the *Detroit Free Press*

1966-70: assistant foreign editor, the *Washington Post*

1970-73: feature writer, the *Washington Post*

1973-79: playing hippie in Colorado and dicking around at trivial jobs like polishing silver in a jewelry store and driving an ice-cream truck (ding-a-ling)

1979: novel *Unnatural Axe* published by Delacorte, a comedy-of-manners about the Colorado counterculture

1981: novel *Driveaway Man* published by Delacorte, about a dreamer who drives his stroke-addled father around the country to snap him out of his lifelong trance

1982-84: columnist (Private Lives), the *Boulder Daily Camera*

1984-2012: magazine feature writer for *Conde Nast Traveler, Travel and Leisure, Outside, GQ, Esquire, Men's Journal, Rolling Stone, Fortune, California, Historic Preservation, American Way,* the *Washington Post,* the *New York Times,* the *Los Angeles Times*

2012: co-author of the e-book *True Tales of an Outback Guide: Why Kangaroos Go Boing-Boing-Boing*